PARASITOLOGY
FOR PARENTS

PARASITOLOGY FOR PARENTS

A Guide for Domestic and Travel
Acquired Parasitic Diseases for Children

Michael W. Simon, MD, PhD

Universal-Publishers
Irvine • Boca Raton

Parasitology for Parents: A Guide for Domestic and Travel Acquired
Parasitic Diseases for Children

Universal Publishers, Inc.
Irvine • Boca Raton
USA • 2025
www.Universal-Publishers.com

ISBN: 978-1-59942-750-8 (pbk.)
ISBN: 978-1-59942-751-5 (ebk.)
ISBN: 978-1-59942-752-2 (aud.)

Typeset by Medlar Publishing Solutions Pvt Ltd, India
Cover design by Ivan Popov

Library of Congress Cataloging-in-Publication Data

Names: Simon, Michael W., 1950- author.
Title: Parasitology for parents : a guide for domestic and travel acquired
    parasitic diseases for children / Michael W. Simon, MD, PhD.
Description: Irvine : Universal Publishers, 2025. | Includes index.
Identifiers: LCCN 2024048515 (print) | LCCN 2024048516 (ebook) |
    ISBN 9781599427508 (pbk) | ISBN 9781599427515 (ebk) |
    ISBN 9781599427522 (aud)
Subjects: LCSH: Parasitic diseases in children--Handbooks, manuals, etc. |
    Medical parasitology--Handbooks, manuals, etc.
Classification: LCC RJ401 .S585 2025 (print) | LCC RJ401 (ebook) |
    DDC 618.92/96--dc23/eng/20250114
LC record available at https://lccn.loc.gov/2024048515
LC ebook record available at https://lccn.loc.gov/2024048516

Table of Contents

Acknowledgement

The author would like to acknowledge the assistance of Henry J. Simon, P.A.-C. for his help in organizing this material and Sarah Miller, B.A. for her assistance in editing this text.

Foreword

This text is a resource that allows you to assess your child's risks of exposure and health consequences of acquiring parasitic infections The goal is to inform parents and those participating in childcare of the risks their children have for and developing symptoms of parasitic illnesses acquired from domestic and travel exposures, recreational and leisure activities and food and beverage consumption. This text also presents prophylactic and preventive measures and the most up-to-date recommended treatment. It has a geographic listing of where different parasites may naturally occur, their life cycle and how they may be acquired. It is divided into sections for easy and quick access.

Sarah Miller, B.A.
October 2024

Parasitology Points

Staying home or traveling to different parts of the world you think are safe . . . . Think again! Even your own backyard and geographic neighbors may be havens for parasitic infections and disease!

Pets should have regular preventive health visits with their veterinarian and be checked for parasites.

Children should never walk barefooted in unpaved grass or soil areas.

Just because you live in a developed country does not mean you are not at risk of acquiring a parasitic disease.

You should never eat undercooked or raw meat whether it be red, white or seafood or raw aquatic plants.

Never eat unwashed food cultivated in soil that is fertilized with human or animal feces.

Think your processed foods are safe, think again! Our foods may be contaminated with rodent feces and insect parts. The FDA recognizes that fly eggs, rodent feces and insect parts are contaminants in our food. The FDA allows a certain level to be present as natural, unavoidable contaminants that occur during growing, processing and packaging of food. The FDA has defined levels of these deemed safe for human consumption.

General Information/ Introduction

Parasites are all around us. They are part of the unseen world we share. We are at risk for acquiring parasitic infections from international and domestic travel, from walking around our own backyard to travel to distant parts of the world. These infections may be acute or chronic, symptom free or cause life-threatening disease.

Think our foods are safe, think again. Eating our daily foods or exotic imported foods puts us at risk for parasitic infections. The FDA allows a certain specified safe amount of rodent and insect parts and feces and other toxic substances in our foods during the natural course of their growth and processing.

Children of all ages and in all countries are at risk of developing parasitic diseases. Parasites are not selective. With the opportunity they will equally infect those of affluence and poverty. The opportunity may be limited by geographic and environmental factors.

A parasite is an organism that will live in or on a host and depends upon that host to provide its food and nutrition. Those in developed and developing countries may acquire a parasitic illness from domestic or international travel. Children who participate in mission trips, international travel as part of a curriculum or for a cultural experience may acquire parasitic infestations or infection that are unique to that area. They may return ill or not develop symptoms for weeks or months.

Be mindful of prophylactic measures recommended by the World Health Organization (WHO) or Centers For Disease Control (CDC). Do your research and be informed of different parasites or pathogens that are prevalent to that area or region of travel. It is important to complete a full course of prophylactic medicine if or as it is recommended by health resources.

Just because you live in a developed country does not mean you are not at risk of acquiring a parasitic infection. Certain infections are more likely diseases of affluence like *Cryptosporidium* from swallowing contaminated water from pools, hot tubs, fountains, rivers, creeks or lakes during recreational activities. Likewise, the brain eating ameba *Naegleria* may be acquired by swimming in contaminated lakes.

Our pets and wild animals may be sources of parasites. It is possible for pets to harbor and pass certain parasites to people. Puppies and kittens are more likely to be infected with roundworms and hookworms. Cat feces may contain *Toxoplasma* which may be spread by contact with contaminated soil or litter boxes. If a pregnant woman is infected with *Toxoplasma*, she may spread the parasite to her baby before birth. Raccoon feces may be a source of *Baylisascaris*.

Children in day care are at risk for *Giardia* and those in school and preschool may become infested with scabies and head lice. Pinworms are a common infestation in children especially those in preschool as well as young school-age children. Food is also an important source of parasitic infections. Sources are undercooked meat, undercooked or raw fish, crabs, mollusks, oysters, food grown in soil that is fertilized with human or animal feces and raw aquatic plants.

Intestinal worm infestations like *Strongyloides* and hookworm, skin disease from cutaneous larva migrans may occur in developed and developing countries. Overall other parasitic diseases may be common but unrecognized in developed countries. They may be more frequent and due to familiarity better recognized in developing countries. This is especially true for Malaria. Children living in Malaria endemic areas particularly African children less than five years of age are at a greater risk of severe Malaria illness and death. Traveling to these areas puts all children at risk for becoming infected with Malaria.

In developing countries, children are at a higher risk due to their play exposure to other types of intestinal worm infestations. By walking barefooted in or ingesting contaminated soil they may acquire hookworm or whipworm infections. Standing or swimming in *Schistosoma* infested water may result in the parasite penetrating the skin and initiating infection. A type of Blackfly through biting may transmit Onchocerisis or Filaria may be spread through mosquito bites. These diseases are "neglected tropical diseases" because due to circumstances and exposure are more likely to affect impoverished people living in developing areas of the world. Travelers to these areas may likewise return to their home and become ill from these parasites.

Parasites may be helminths (worms), protozoa and ectoparasites. There are specific helminths that are of concern because they produce illness in people. They have a complex lifecycle involving different stages. In people, they are taken in at a specific stage and mature into an adult in the human body. The adult does not multiply in the human body. There are three types of helminths, trematodes (flatworms), cestodes (tapeworms), and nematodes (roundworms). They are spread by different stages passing through contaminated feces in the soil or water then back to a human by oral ingestion (fecal-oral route). Sometimes stages must pass through an "intermediate host" before reaching a stage that may infect people.

Protozoa are one celled, microscopic organisms that may be parasitic or free living. As parasites they multiply in humans which result in illness. They may live in the human intestine, blood stream, tissues or organs. They may be transmitted through the bite of certain types of mosquitoes or flies. Those living in the gastrointestinal tract may be spread by ingesting food or water contaminated with feces containing protozoans or by person-to-person contact.

Ectoparasites like mites, fleas and ticks attach or burrow into the skin and survive for weeks to months. Through their biting and feeding they may transmit different microorganisms that cause significant disease, Lyme disease and Rocky Mountain Spotted Fever just to name a few. Developed and developing areas of the world including the North Midwestern and Northeastern states in the United States have *Babesia*, a Malaria like parasite carried by ticks. Likewise, *Giardia*, *Cryptosporidium* and *Cyclospora* are protozoa that may cause diarrhea, skin sores, cough, muscle aches and in severe cases weight loss, malnutrition and neurological symptoms. Drinking water contaminated with infectious feces may result in Amebic Dysentery or Guinea Worm disease.

The goal of this text is to inform parents of the risks their children have for acquiring and developing symptoms associated with parasitic illnesses from domestic and travel exposures as well as prophylactic and preventive measures and the most up to date recommended treatment.

Index: Geographic Location of Parasites

Africa:
African Eye Worm. Amebic meningoencephalitis. Brain cyst. Cysticercosis. Dwarf tapeworm. *Endolimax. Entamoeba.* Hookworm. *Hymenolepis.* Liver fluke. Lung Fluke. Neurocysticercosis. Rat tapeworm. Roundworm. Round worm of dogs. Roundworm of cats. *Schistosoma. Toxocara.* Whipworm.

Central Africa: African eye worm. Sleeping sickness. *Trypanosoma.*

East Africa: *Echinococcus.* Hydatid disease. Sleeping sickness. *Trypanosoma.*

North Africa: *Echinococcus.* Elephantiasis. Filaria. Hydatid disease. Kala azar. *Leishmania.*

Northeast Africa: *Echinococcus.* Hydatid disease.

Sub-Saharan Africa: Asian tapeworm. *Ascaris.* Guinea Worm. Hookworm. Malaria. *Plasmodium.* Pork tapeworm. *Strongyloides.* Tapeworm. *Toxoplasma.*

West Africa: African Eye Worm. Sleeping sickness. *Trypanosoma.*

Afghanistan:
Dwarf tapeworm. *Hymenolepis.* Kala azar. *Leishmania.* Rat tapeworm.

Alor:
Elephantiasis. Filariasis.

America:
Chagas disease. *Dientamoeba. Dipylidium.* Dog tapeworm. Dwarf tapeworm. *Enterobius. Giardia.* Hookworm. *Hymenolepis.* Malaria. Pinworms. *Plasmodium.* Rat tapeworm, Roundworm. Roundworm of dogs. Roundworm of cats. *Strongloides.* Tapeworm. *Toxocara. Toxoplasma. Trichinella. Trypanosoma.*

Atlantic Coast States: *Dirofilaria.* Dog heartworm.

Cape Cod to Eastern Long Island, Shelter Island, Nantucket, Martha's Vineyard: *Babesia.*

Gulf Coast States: Dog heartworm. *Dirofilaria.*

Midwestern States: *Babesia. Toxoplasma.*

Mississippi River Basin: *Dirofilaria.* Dog heartworm. Lung fluke.

Northern: Amebic meningoencephalitis.

Northeastern States: *Babesia.*

Southeastern States: Amebic meningoencephalitis. *Strongyloides. Trichinella.*

Southern States: Amebic meningoencephalitis. Chagas disease. Lung fluke. *Toxoplasma. Trypanosoma.*

Southwestern states: Amebic meningoencephalitis.

Western: Chagas disease. *Toxoplasma. Trypanosoma.*

Alaska: Broad fish tapeworm. Diphyllobothrium. Echinococcus.

Arizona: Amebic meningoencephalitis. *Echinococcus.* Hydatid disease.

Arkansas: Amebic meningoencephalitis. *Babesia.*

California: Amebic meningoencephalitis. *Babesia.* Chagas disease. *Echinococcus.* Granulomatous amebic encephalopathy. Hydatid disease. *Trypanosoma.*

Connecticut: *Babesia.*

Delaware: *Babesia.*

Florida: Amebic meningoencephalitis. Malaria. *Plasmodium.*

Georgia: Granulomatous amebic encephalopathy.

Hawaii: *Heterophyes.*

Indiana: Amebic meningoencephalitis.

Iowa: *Trichinella.*

Kansas: Amebic meningoencephalitis.

Kentucky: *Babesia. Strongyloides. Trichinella.*

Louisiana: Chagas disease. *Trypanosoma.*

Maine: *Babesia.*

Maryland: Amebic meningoencephalitis. *Babesia.* Malaria. *Plasmodium.*

Michigan: *Babesia.*

Minnesota: Amebic meningoencephalitis. *Babesia.*

Nebraska: Amebic meningoencephalitis.

New Hampshire: *Babesia.*

New Jersey: *Babesia.*

New Mexico: *Echinococcus.* Hydatid disease.

New York: *Babesia.* Granulomatous amebic encephalopathy.

Oklahoma: Amebic meningoencephalitis.

Oregon: *Cryptosporidium.*

Pennsylvania: *Babesia.*

South Carolina: Amebic meningoencephalitis.

Tennessee: Chagas disease. *Trypanosoma.*

Texas: Amebic meningoencephalitis. Chagas disease. *Dirofilaria.* Dog heartworm. Granulomatous amebic encephalopathy. *Heterophytes.* Malaria. *Plasmodium. Trypanosoma.*

Utah: *Echinococcus.* Hydatid disease

Vermont: *Babesia.*

Virginia: Amebic meningoencephalitis. *Babesia.*

Washington DC: *Babesia.*

Wyoming: Amebic meningoencephalitis.

Wisconsin: *Cryptosporidium*.

Americas:
Ascaris. Asian tapeworm. *Dipylidium*. Dog tapeworm. Dwarf tapeworm. *Echinostoma*. Elephantiasis. *Hymenolepis*. Lung fluke. Pork tapeworm. Rat tapeworm, Roundworm of dogs. Roundworm of cats. Whipworm.

Angola:
Plains of Northern Angola: African Eye Worm. Guinea worm.

Argentina:
Dipylidium. Dog tapeworm. Dwarf tapeworm. *Echinococcus*. *Echinostoma*. Hookworm. Hydatid disease. *Hymenolepis*. Rat tapeworm. Roundworm. Roundworm of dogs. Roundworm of cats. *Trichinella*. *Toxocara*.

Asia:
Amebic meningoencephalitis. *Ascaris*. Asian tapeworm. *Dipylidium*. *Dirofilaria*. Dog heartworm. Dog tapeworm. Dwarf tapeworm. *Echinococcus*. *Echinostoma*. *Endolimax*. Guinea Worm. Hydatid disease. *Hymenolepis*. Kala azar. *Leishmania*. Liver fluke. Lung fluke. Pork tapeworm. Rat tapeworm, Roundworm of dogs. Roundworm of cats. Tapeworm. *Toxocara*. *Trichuris*. Whipworm.

Central Asia: *Echinococcus*. Hydatid disease.

East Asia: Chinese liver fluke. *Clonorchis*. Hookworm. Oriental liver fluke

Mekong basin. Chinese liver fluke. *Opisthorchis*. Oriental liver fluke

Southeast Asia: Brain cyst. Cysticercosis. Elephantiasis. Filariasis. Malaria. Neurocysticercosis. *Plasmodium*. Roundworm. Roundworm of dogs. Roundworm of cats. *Schistosoma*. *Strongyloides*. *Toxocara*.

Australia:
Amebic meningoencephalitis. *Babesia*. *Dientamoeba*. *Dipylidium*. *Dirofilaria*. Dog heartworm. Dog tapeworm. *Echinococcus*. *Endolimax*. Hookworm. Hydatid disease. *Toxoplasma*.

Northern Australia: Hookworm.

Balkans:
Heterophyes.

Bangladesh:
Dwarf tapeworm. Hookworm. *Hymenolepis.* Kala azar. *Leishmania.* Liver fluke, Rat tapeworm.

Belgium:
Dientamoeba. Hookworm.

Benin (Southeastern):
African Eye Worm.

Bolivia:
Babesia. Chagas disease. Liver fluke. *Trichinella. Trypanosoma.*

Borneo:
Malaria. *Plasmodium.*

Brazil:
Brain cyst. Cysticercosis. Dipylidium. Dog tapeworm. Dwarf tapeworm. *Echinococcus. Endolimax.* Espundia. Hydatid disease. *Hymenolepis. Leishmania.* Liver fluke. Neurocysticercosis. River blindness. Rat tapeworm. Roundworm. Roundworm of dogs. Roundworm of cats. *Schistosoma. Toxocara. Toxoplasma.*

British Isles:
Dientamoeba.

Bulgaria:
Dipylidium. Dog Tapeworm.

Byelorussia:
Chinese liver fluke. Opisthorchis. Oriental Liver Fluke.

Cambodia:
Chinese liver fluke. *Echinostoma. Opisthorchis.* Oriental liver fluke. *Schistosoma. Strongyloides. Trichinella.*

Cameroon:
African eye worm. Lung fluke. River blindness.

Canary Islands:
Babesia.

Canada:
Broad fish tapeworm. *Dientamoeba. Dipylidium. Diphyllobothrium. Dirofilaria.* Dog heartworm. Dog tapeworm. Dwarf tapeworm. *Echinococcus.* Hydatid disease. *Hymenolepis.* Lung fluke. Rat tapeworm.

Caribbean:
Hookworm. Liver fluke. *Schistosoma.*

Central African Republic:
African eye worm. River blindness.

Central America:
Brain cyst. Chagas disease. Cysticercosis. Elephantiasis. Entamoeba. Espundia. Filariasis. Hookworm. *Leishmania.* Neurocysticercosis. Pork tapeworm. Tapeworm. *Toxoplasma. Trypanosoma.*

Chad:
African eye worm. Guinea worm.

Chile:
Broad fish tapeworm. *Dipylidium. Diphyllobothrium.* Dog tapeworm. *Echinococcus.* Hydatid disease. Liver fluke.

China:
Asian tapeworm. *Babesia.* Brain cyst. Broad fish tapeworm Chinese liver fluke. *Clonorchis.* Cysticercosis. *Dipylidium.* Dog tapeworm. *Echinococcus. Echinostoma. Heterophyes.* Hookworm. Hydatid disease. Liver fluke. Lung fluke. Neurocysticercosis. *Opisthorchis.* Oriental liver fluke. Roundworm. Roundworm of dogs. Roundworm of cats. *Schistosoma.* Tapeworm. *Toxocara. Trichinella.*

Mainland: *Babesia.*

Northeastern: *Babesia.*

South: Hookworm.

Southern: hookworm. *Schistosoma.*

Western: *Echinococcus.* Hydatid disease.

Columbia:
Babesia. Chagas disease. *Trypanosoma.*

Corsica:
Schistosoma.

Costa Rica:
Dwarf tapeworm. *Hymenolepis.* Rat tapeworm.

Cote d Ivory:
Endolimax. Kala azar. *Schistosoma.*

Democratic Republic of Congo:
African eye worm. *Babesia.* Chagas disease. River blindness. *Trypanosoma.*

Denmark:
Babesia.

Dominican Republic:
Schistosoma.

Eastern Mediterranean:
Dwarf tapeworm. *Hymenolepis.* Rat tapeworm.

Ecuador:
Brain cyst. Cysticercosis. Lung fluke. Neurocysticercosis.

Egypt:
Babesia. Dwarf tapeworm. Hookworm. *Hymenolepis.* Liver fluke. Rat tapeworm. *Schistosoma.*

El Salvador:
Hookworm.

England:
Amebic meningoencephalitis. *Dipylidium*. Dog tapeworm.

Ethiopia:
Dwarf tapeworm. Guinea worm. *Hymenolepis*. Kala azar. *Leishmania*. Rat tapeworm.

Europe:
Amebic meningoencephalitis. Broad fish tapeworm. *Dientamoeba*. *Dipylidium*. *Diphyllobothrium*. Dog tapeworm. Dwarf tapeworm. *Echinostoma*. *Endolimax*. *Hymenolepis*. Rat tapeworm. Roundworm. Roundworm of dogs. Roundworm of cats. *Strongyloides*. *Toxocara*.

Eastern Europe: Chinese liver fluke. *Clonorchis*. Pork tapeworm. *Opisthorchis*. Oriental liver fluke. Tapeworm.

Southern Europe: Kala azar. *Leishmania*.

Southwestern Europe: *Echinococcus*. Hydatid disease.

France:
Babesia. Broad fish tapeworm. *Diphyllobothrium*. *Dirofilaria*. Dog heartworm. Roundworm. Roundworm of dogs. Roundworm of cat. *Toxocara*. *Toxoplasma*. *Trichinella*.

Finland:
Broad fish tapeworm. *Diphyllobothrium*.

French Guiana:
Toxoplasma.

Gabon:
African Eye Worm.

Germany:
Babesia. Chinese liver fluke. *Dipylidium*. Dog tapeworm. *Endolimax*. Hookworm. *Opisthorchis*. Oriental liver fluke.

Ghana:
Guinea worm.

Greece:
Chinese liver fluke. *Dirofilaria*. Dog heartworm. Oriental liver fluke. *Opisthorchis*.

Guadeloupe:
Schistosoma.

Guatemala:
Brain cyst. Cysticercosis. *Dipylidium*. Dog tapeworm. Neurocysticercosis.

Guinea, Equatorial:
African Eye Worm.

Guyana:
Toxoplasma.

Honduras:
Brain cyst. Cysticercosis. Hookworm. Neurocysticercosis.

India:
Amebic meningoencephalitis. Asian tapeworm. *Babesia*. Brain cyst. Cysticercosis. *Dipylidium*. Dog tapeworm. Dwarf tapeworm. *Echinostoma*. Elephantiasis. *Entamoeba*. Filariasis. *Heterophyes*. Hookworm. *Hymenolepis*. Kala azar. *Leishmania*. Liver fluke. Lung fluke. Neurocysticercosis. Pork tapeworm. Rat tapeworm. Roundworm. Roundworm of dog. Roundworm of cat. Tapeworm. *Toxocara*.

Indonesia:
Asian tapeworm. *Echinostoma*. Liver fluke. *Schistosoma*. Tapeworm.

Iran:
Granulomatous amebic encephalopathy. *Heterophyes*. Kala azar. *Leishmania*. Liver fluke. *Schistosoma*.

Iraq:
Schistosoma.

Israel:
Amebic meningoencephalitis. *Dientamoeba*. *Heterophyes*.

Italy:
Broad fish tapeworm. *Dientamoeba. Dipylidium. Diphyllobothrium. Dirofilaria.* Dog heartworm. Dog tapeworm. Chinese liver fluke. *Opisthorchis.* Oriental liver fluke. *Trichinella.*

Ivory Coast:
Babesia.

Japan:
Asian tapeworm. *Babesia.* Broad fish tapeworm. Chinese liver fluke. *Clonorchis. Dipylidium. Diphyllobothrium.* Dog tapeworm. Filariasis. *Heterophyes.* Lung fluke. Oriental liver fluke. Roundworm. Roundworm of dog. Roundworm of cat. Tapeworm. *Toxocara. Trichinella.*

Kenya:
Echinostoma. Schistosoma.

Korea:
Asian tapeworm. Broad fish tapeworm. *Diphyllobothrium.* Filariasis. *Heterophyes.* Roundworm. Roundworm of dog. Roundworm of cat. Tapeworm. *Toxocara.*

Lao People's Democratic Republic:
Asian tapeworm. Chinese liver fluke. Dwarf tapeworm. *Echinostoma. Heterophyes. Hymenolepis.* Liver fluke. Lung fluke. *Opisthorchis.* Oriental liver fluke. Rat tapeworm, *Schistosoma. Strongyloides.* Tapeworm.

Latin America:
Amebic meningoencephalitis. Brain cyst. Cysticercosis. Dwarf tapeworm, Elephantiasis. Filariasis. *Hymenolepis.* Malaria. Neurocysticercosis. *Plasmodium.* Pork tapeworm. Rat tapeworm. *Strongyloides.* Tapeworm. *Toxoplasma.*

Latvia: Granulomatous amebic encephalopathy.

Lebadon:
Trichinella.

Lembata:
Filariasis.

Liberia:
Lung fluke.

Malawi:
Sleeping sickness. *Trypanosoma*.

Malaysia:
Echinostoma. Liver fluke. Malaria. *Plasmodium*. *Toxoplasma*.

Mali:
Guinea worm. *Schistosoma*.

Mallorca:
Schistosoma.

Manchuria:
Chinese liver fluke. *Clonorchis*. *Heterophyes*. Oriental liver fluke.

Martinque:
Schistosoma.

Mediterranean region:
Echinococcus. Hydatid disease.

Mexico:
Amebic meningoencephalitis. *Babesia*. Brain cyst. Chagas disease. Cysticercosis. *Dipylidium*. Dog tapeworm. Dwarf tapeworm, *Entamoeba*. Granulomatous amebic encephalopathy. *Heterophyes*. *Hymenolepis*. Liver fluke. Neurocysticercosis. Pork tapeworm. Rat tapeworm. Roundworm. Roundworm of dog. Roundworm of cat. Tapeworm. *Toxocara*. *Trichinella*. *Trypanosoma*.

Middle East:
Kala azar. *Leishmania*. *Schistosoma*.

Mozambique:
Babesia.

Myanmar:
Malaria. *Plasmodium*.

Nepal:
Asian tapeworm. Brain cyst. Cysticercosis. *Echinostoma*. *Heterophyes*. Liver fluke. Neurocysticercosis. Tapeworm.

Netherlands:
Babesia. *Dientamoeba*. Liver fluke.

New Guinea:
Lung fluke. *Trichinella*.

New Zealand:
Amebic meningoencephalitis. Broad fish tapeworm. *Diphyllobothrium*.

Nicaragua:
Endolimax.

Nigeria:
Amebic meningoencephalitis. African Eye Worm. Guinea Worm. Lung fluke. Roundworm. Roundworm of dog. Roundworm of cat. *Schistosoma*. *Toxocara*.

Nile Delta:
Heterophyes.

Nile River Valley:
Schistosoma.

North America:
Chinese liver fluke. *Echinostoma*. *Endolimax*. Liver fluke. Lung fluke. *Opisthorchis*. Oriental Liver Fluke. Pinworms. Pork tapeworm.

Great Lakes area:
Broad fish tapeworm. *Diphyllobothrium*.

Norway:
Babesia.

Oceana:
Echinostoma. Malaria. *Plasmodium*. Pork tapeworm. Tapeworm.

Pacific Islands:
Elephantiasis. Hookworm.

Pakistan:
Amebic meningoencephalitis. *Hymenolepis*. Liver fluke.

Panta:
Filariasis.

Paraguay:
Hookworm.

Peru:
Brain cyst. Broad fish tapeworm. Cysticercosis. *Diphyllobothrium*. Dwarf tapeworm. *Echinococcus*. Espundia. Hookworm. Hydatid disease. *Hymenolepis*. *Leishmania*. Liver fluke. Lung fluke. Neurocysticercosis, Rat tapeworm.

Philippines:
Asian tapeworm. *Dipylidium*. Dog tapeworm. *Echinostoma*. *Heterophyes*. Filariasis. Lung fluke. Malaria. *Plasmodium*. Pork tapeworm. *Schistosoma*. Tapeworm.

Poland:
Dipylidium. Dog tapeworm. *Toxoplasma*. *Trichinella*.

Portugal:
Dientamoeba. Liver fluke.

Puerto Rico:
Dipylidium. Dog tapeworm. *Echinostoma*.

Romania:
Dipylidium. Dog tapeworm. *Trichinella*.

Russia:
Broad fish tapeworm. Chinese liver fluke. *Diphyllobothrium*. *Heterophyes*. Hookworm. Oriental liver fluke. Pork tapeworm. Tapeworm.

Eastern Russia: *Clonorchis*.

Rwanda:
Brain cyst. Cysticercosis. Neurocysticercosis.

Part two geographic location of parasites

Saint Lucia:
Schistosoma.

Samoa:
Elephantiasis. Filariasis.

Saudi Arabia:
Kala azar. *Leishmania. Schistosoma.*

Siberia:
Broadfish tapeworm. Chinese liver fluke. *Diphyllobothrium. Heterophyes. Opisthorchis.* Oriental liver fluke.

Singapore:
Malaria. *Plasmodium.*

South Africa:
Babesia. Broad fish tapeworm. *Dipylidium. Diphyllobothrium.* Dog tapeworm. Roundworm. Roundworm of dog. Roundworm of cat. *Toxocara.*

South America:
Entamoeba. Espundia. Filariasis. Hookworm. *Leishmania.* Lung fluke. Pork tapeworm. Tapeworm.

Pacific Coast: Brain cyst. Broad fish tapeworm. Cysticercosis. *Diphyllobothrium. Echinococcus. Endolimax.* Hookworm. Neurocysticercosis. *Schistosoma.*

South Korea:
Broad fish tapeworm. Chinese Liver fluke. *Clonorchis. Diphyllobothrium. Echinostoma. Opisthorchis.* Oriental Liver Fluke.

South Pacific:
Elephantiasis. Filariasis. Hookworm.

Spain:
Chagas disease. *Dientamoeba. Dipylidium. Dirofilaria.* Dog heartworm. Dog tapeworm. *Heterophyes.* Roundworm. Roundworm of dog. Roundworm of cat. *Strongyloides. Toxocara. Trypanosoma.*

Sri Lanka:
Dipylidium. Dog tapeworm. *Heterophyes.* Hookworm.

Sudan:
African eye worm. *Babesia.* Dwarf tapeworm. Guinea worm. *Heterophyes. Hymenolepis.* Kala azar. *Leishmania.* Rat tapeworm. River blindness. *Schistosoma.*

Sumba:
Filariasis.

Sunda Archipelago:
Filariasis.

Suriname:
Schistosoma.

Sweden:
Dientamoeba. Trypanosoma.

Syria:
Kala azar. *Leishmania.*

Taiwan:
Asian tapeworm. *Babesia.* Broad fish tapeworm. *Diphyllobothrium. Echinostoma. Heterophyes.* Liver fluke. Lung fluke. Tapeworm. *Trichinella.*

Tanzania:
Echinostoma. Trichinella.

Thailand:
Asian tapeworm. Chinese liver fluke. *Clonorchis. Echinostoma. Heterophyes.* Liver fluke. Lung fluke. Malaria. *Opisthorchis.* Oriental liver fluke. *Plasmodium. Strongyloides.* Tapeworm. *Trichinella.*

Timor:
Filariasis.

Tropics:
Elephantiasis. Espundia. *Leishmania.*

Tunisia:
Heterophyes. Roundworm. Roundworm of dog. Roundworm of cat. *Toxocara.*

Turkey:
Dientamoeba. Dipylidium. Dog tapeworm. *Heterophyes.* Kala azar. *Leishmania.*
Liver fluke. *Trichinella.*

Uganda:
African Eye Worm. *Schistosoma.* Sleeping sickness. *Trypanosoma.*

Ukraine:
Chinese liver fluke. *Opisthorchis.* Oriental liver fluke.

Venezuela:
Chagas disease. Lung fluke. River blindness. *Schistosoma. Trypanosoma.*

Vietnam:
Chinese liver fluke. *Clonorchis. Echinostoma.* Hookworm. Liver fluke. Lung
fluke. *Opisthorchis.* Oriental liver fluke. Tapeworm. *Trichinella.*

Virgin Islands: Amebic meningoencephalitis.

Western Hemisphere:
Dirofilaria. Dog heartworm.

West Indies:
Elephantiasis.

Worldwide distribution:
Amebic meningoencephalitis. Broadfish tapeworm. *Diphyllobothrium.*
Chinese liver fluke. *Clonorchis. Cryptosporidium. Dientamoeba. Echinococcus.*
Echinostoma. Endolimax. Entamoeba. Enterobius. Espundia. *Fasciola. Giardia.*

Granulomatous amebic encephalopathy. Hookworm. Hydatid disease. Kala azar. *Leishmania*. Liver fluke. Lung fluke. *Opisthorchis*. Oriental liver fluke. Pinworms. Roundworm. Roundworm of dog. Roundworm of cat. Tapeworm. *Toxocara*. *Toxoplasma*. *Trichinella*. Whipworm.

Yemen:
River blindness. *Schistosoma*.

Yugoslavia:
Babesia.

Zambia:
Brain cyst. Cysticercosis. Neurocysticercosis. Sleeping sickness. *Trypanosoma*.

Zimbabwe:
Schistosoma.

This is the most accurate information available at the time of this text preparation.

What is a Parasite?

Parasitism is a type of symbiosis or living together where one organism lives and survives at the expense of another organism. With parasitism one partner benefits (the parasite), the other partner (the host) does not. It is like relatives coming to visit with you and then you cannot get them to leave. The parasite may live in (endoparasite) or on (ectoparasite) the host and depends on that partner for its nutrition and development. The host also provides a safe, hospitable environment. The parasite lives off the host and gives nothing in return. That does sound like relatives.

Parasites have adapted to invade and live in cells and tissues of their host. Unlike relatives, parasites will be in or on our body and we may not be aware of their presence. They may in many cases produce no or few symptoms unless there are a large number at one time or are overly aggressive and injurious to the host. We may acquire parasites by walking around outdoors without shoes and socks, through insect bites, eating raw meats, fruits and vegetables, drinking dirty water or poor hand hygiene, that is not washing hands regularly.

Parasites require their passage through specific hosts generally in a specific sequence to continue their life cycle. People may not be the host of choice and become accidentally infected, an accidental host. People may develop symptoms but not allow the parasite to complete its lifecycle, a dead end for the parasite. To be effective, parasites must be successful in evading and escaping the attention of their host's immune system.

Types of Parasites

Parasites may be helminths (worms), protozoa or ectoparasites.

There are three types of helminths, cestodes (tapeworms), nematodes (roundworms) and trematodes (flatworms). Cestodes are tapeworms which means they are ribbon shaped with many body segments and a distinctive head. They are parasites of the intestinal tract where they attach to the lining of the intestines. The terminal, last end segment of the adult worm undergoes maturation and may contain hundreds to thousands of eggs. This last segment will detach and pass in the feces into the environment. Eggs are then taken in by the next host which may be different types of warm-blooded animals and fish. This is the next step in the tapeworm's lifecycle. In these hosts, larval forms may be in their body tissues or organs. People will acquire the larval form by eating contaminated raw or undercooked meat, fish and grains. The larvae will continue the lifecycle and mature into adults.

Nematodes are roundworms, they are shaped like earthworms. There are many different nematodes with only a few maladapting into a parasitic existence. They become dependent on a specific requirement for particular hosts. They cannot survive independently without this host which is needed for their survival and completing their lifecycle. People, especially children, may become infected with a large number of a single type or multiple types of nematodes affecting their health and well-being. Adult nematodes will produce and release eggs which go through a specific sequence and hosts for development into new roundworms.

Trematodes are flatworms or flukes. They have a flattened body. They have a worldwide distribution and are found anywhere where there are untreated human feces, especially when it is used as a fertilizer. Those that infect humans are found in specific regions across the globe. Forms and stages of the parasite will live in the tissues, lungs, intestinal tract and blood of their host.

Their lifecycle requires at least two different hosts. Eggs are produced and released into the environment. There they will hatch or be ingested by the next host, usually a snail. Their development continues producing the infectious stage which may be released in freshwater or in the body of cold-blooded vertebrates like fish, crustaceans and clams. People will become infected by eating undercooked fish, crabs and frogs as well as unwashed contaminated vegetation like water caltrops.

Protozoans are one-celled microscopic animals. They may be free-living or parasitic. They have a worldwide distribution and have adapted to live in cells and tissues of other organisms. They are a diverse group and will vary from a simple to complex lifecycle and have adapted to infecting animals of all types including humans. Those infecting humans have adapted to live in the intestinal tract, bloodstream, tissues and other organs. Because they produce disease and death in a diverse group of hosts, they have made certain areas of the world uninhabitable through their effect on the health and well-being of people and their livestock. Protozoans characteristically have an active feeding stage called a trophozoite and some have a resting stage, Oocyst that is resistant to changing and harsh environmental conditions. Infection will occur through ingesting the cystic form. As parasites they multiply in humans which result in illness. They may be transmitted through the bite of certain types of mosquitoes and flies. Those living in the gastrointestinal tract may be spread by ingestion of food or water contaminated with feces containing protozoans or by direct person-to-person contact.

Ectoparasites are mites, fleas and ticks that attach or burrow into the skin and survive for weeks to months. Through their biting and feeding they may transmit different microorganisms that cause significant disease.

Pet Related Illnesses and Infections

This section is included because pets are an important source of infection for children. It is not limited to parasites that may be passed from pets but provides information regarding different germs and illnesses that pets may spread to their human contacts. In many homes pets are an important part of the family and are even treated as family members. This is especially true for dogs, less so for cats. Dogs were the first animal to be domesticated. Worldwide estimates are that there are around 900 million domesticated dogs. Of these 20 to 30% are companion pets while the others are free roaming. Pets may add both pleasure, companionship and responsibility for children. Pets are unfortunately also a common source of germs producing illness and disease in children. Pets may be traditional, dogs and cats, or nontraditional, exotic pets, reptiles, amphibians, certain types of small mammals and wildlife. The recent statistics are staggering for the number of homes in the United States having both traditional and non-traditional pets.

84.9 million households have pets with 67% of all homes having at least one pet.
63.4 million households have a dog.
42.7 million households have a cat.
11.5 million households have freshwater fish.
5.7 million households have a bird.
5.4 million households have small animals (hamsters, gerbils, guinea pigs, ferrets, rabbits, mice, rats).
4.5 million households have reptiles (lizards, snakes, turtles).
1.6 million households have horses.
1.6 million households have saltwater fish.

Children less than five years of age are at the greatest risk of becoming ill because of poor hygiene and their natural attraction to animals. They are more likely to have direct contact through the animals' saliva through licking and biting, scratches, sneezing, coughing, handling the animal or fleas from the infected animal. The animals are most likely to be symptom-free at the time of exposure. Children may also acquire germs through contaminated animal feces in the environment, food or water. These illnesses may be from bacteria, viruses, fungi or parasites.

More than 4 million dog bites causing a wound or puncture injury occur in the United States each year. Most bites occur from a family's own pet and generally are on the hands or face. The bite may introduce a mixture of germs from the dog's saliva most often *Pasteurella* and *Staphylococcus*. To minimize infection the wound should be cleaned with an antibacterial soap and antiseptic like peroxide. Although fewer than 20% of bites may still become infected, a healthcare provider should evaluate every bite as soon as possible. Oral and topical antibiotics may initially be prescribed to prevent infection or to treat infection that has already become established. If the infection is severe, a shot or intravenous antibiotic may be needed.

There are fewer cat bites, with an estimated 500,000 cat bites in the United States each year. Most cat bites occur on the hands and are "puncture" wounds from their teeth. There may be lacerations from the cat teeth or cat claw scratches. Cat teeth are more pointed producing deeper puncture wounds which are more likely to cause soft-tissue abscesses. Cats may carry *Pasteurella*, *Staphylococcus* and *Streptococcus* in their saliva. They may also harbor a germ called *Bartonella* which may produce Cat Scratch Fever. The recommendations for wound care are the same as for dog bites. Initial cleansing and disinfection of the wound and seeing a healthcare provider for additional recommendations and care.

Germs, illnesses and infections spread by specific animals:
Dogs and cats: *Giardia, Isopora, Trichuris, Toxocara, Echinococcus, Cryptosporidium, Toxoplasma, Campylobacter, Helicobacter, Francisella, Dypilidium, Opisthorchis,* Q fever, Rabies. cat and dog *Bordetella* (kennel cough). In dog urine, *Leptospira* and *Brucella.* Canine scabies/mange from contact with fur. Lyme disease, *Bartonella,* Babesiosis, Ehrlichiosis from ticks on dogs. Cats may carry *Microsporum* which may cause Ringworm in people and other fungi which may cause patchy hair loss for people. Cat scabies caused by mites may also spread to people.

Small animals and mammals: *Salmonella, Yersinia* (Plague), Rabies, *Escherichia coli, Salmonella, Pasteurella, Cryptosporidium, Campylobacter*, Raccoon variant Rabies, *Spirillum* (Rat Bite Fever), Lymphocytic Choriomeningitis Virus.

Fish and aquatic animals: *Salmonella*, skin infections with *Erysipelothrix*, non-group A *Streptococcus* and *Mycobacterium*.

Chickens and baby poultry: *Salmonella*.

Reptiles and amphibians: *Salmonella, Shigella, Vibrio*, frozen rodents sold as reptile food may have *Salmonella*.

Birds: *Salmonella, Giardia, Campylobacter, Cryptococcus, Pasteurella, Mycobacterium, Chlamydia*/Psittacosis, mites, Bird Influenza strains and both *Histoplasma* and *Cryptococcus* from bird droppings.

Farm animals and petting zoos: Escherichia coli, Salmonella, Cryptosporidium.

Non-human primates: Hepatitis A, Hepatitis B, Monkeypox, *Salmonella, Shigella, Campylobacter*, Ameba, *Strongyloides, Giardia, Yersinia*, Herpes virus simiae (brain inflammation).

Preventive measures include keeping pets healthy with regular veterinarian checkups, vaccinations and free of intestinal parasites, ticks, fleas, lice and mites. There should be effective measures for flea and tick control. Remove cat and dog hair or dander from surfaces, furniture, carpets and bedding. Properly, safely discard any animal feces. Hands should be properly washed after handling pets. Do not let pets lick on children or other companions. Keep pets safe and monitored. Do not let them drink surface or toilet water or interact with wild animals. Keep pets away from areas where food is prepared. Teach children safety measures when around animals and to avoid wild, stray or unknown animals even if they seem friendly.

Parasitic Risks for International and Domestic Adoptions

Adopted children present a special population with unique needs. They may have congenital birth defects or other disorders. Their special needs may be the result of exposure to infectious diseases before or after birth, malnutrition, emotional or physical abuse or neglect. Of special interest is the concern that they may be infected with parasites. This may be correlated with their age at adoption and length of time living in an orphanage or foster care.

Estimates for international adoptions project that there is a 15 up to 47% rate of parasitic infection with 10% having more than one parasite. The continent where the child resided is associated with the prevalence and the specific parasite producing the infection. The most commonly reported parasites are *Giardia, Schistosoma, Toxocara* and *Strongyloides*. However, of these the most frequently recovered parasite is *Giardia* recovered in as many as 19% of internationally adopted children. Their diagnosis may be further confused, delayed or complicated by as many as 50% of these children with parasitic infection having no symptoms.

Essentially any parasite reviewed in this text may be a parasite of interest for any international adoptee. Those adopted domestically are still at risk for a parasitic infection depending upon the area of their residence. Newborns adopted internationally and domestically have a much lower risk of parasitic infections. The Centers for Disease Control (CDC), World Health Organization (WHO) and this text may provide information about parasites that a child may acquire from specific geographic areas. There is an observation that the earlier a child has a parasitic infection, they are at a greater risk to develop anxiety, depression or a learning disorder later in life.

Recommended testing for an adopted child at risk would include a complete blood count looking for an elevated number of eosinophils, elevated total IgE level in blood, visual evidence of parasites in a stool, blood or tissue sample and for a specific parasite measuring antibody or nucleic material via PCR test from a blood, tissue or stool sample. The diagnosis and treatment of each parasite is reviewed and discussed in this text.

African Eye Worm

Loiasis
Loa loa

Loa loa is a filaria nematode also known as African Eye worm. It is spread by feeding of the infected female biting deer fly also called horsefly. It is estimated there are 3 to 13 million people infected with *Loa loa*. Forest exposure and the number of infected flies in an area affect the occurrence of *Loa loa*. It occurs in ecological areas of deer or horsefly habitat range including the rain forest of West and Central Africa, Southeastern Benin, Cameroon, coastal plains of northern Angola, Chad, Equatorial Guinea, Central Africa Republic, Sudan, Nigeria, Gabon, Uganda and the Democratic Republic of Congo.

The horsefly or deer fly lives and breeds in rain forest and lays their eggs in muddy swamps. These flies are daytime feeders and are attracted to movement. When an infected bite occurs, it deposits the L3 larvae onto the skin. These larvae then enter the bite site. Over the next three months they mature into adult worms. They live in the subcutaneous tissue and may migrate any-where in the body including under the subconjunctiva, outer layer of the eyeball. After 3 to 9 months the adult worms start to produce thousands of microfilariae that pass into the lungs and from there they are released into the bloodstream and back to the skin. They are ingested by the feeding female horsefly or deer flies. Over the next 10 to 12 days in the flies, the micro-filariae transform into the L3 infective larval stage. During this time, they pass from the fly midgut to the chest muscles and eventually to the feeding apparatus, the proboscis. Then they are passed back to people by fly feeding completing the lifecycle. Adult worms may live up to 20 years. They do not produce additional adult worms. Adults come only from the development of the infective L3 larva in infected people.

Infection occurs only in those who live or visit endemic areas. Infection requires recurrent or chronic feeding by infected flies over weeks to years.

Most infections remain asymptomatic. There will be transient localized sub-cutaneous skin swelling known as Calabar swelling. Migration of the adult worms may occur across the subconjunctiva of the eye. These are the two features of this infection. With first time exposure to *Loa loa*, there may be allergic type symptoms with hives, itching and wheezing. The swelling is the result of the body's reaction to the movement of the adult worms or release of the microfilariae. These symptoms are most likely to occur with the initial infection. Swelling may occur anywhere but is most pronounced on the face and extremities. Pain and itching may occur before swelling develops. Swelling may last for several days to several weeks.

The adult worm may migrate to the eye and pass under the outer layer of the eyeball. The worm may be visualized at this time taking up to 10 to 20 minutes to traverse the eye, hence the name "African Eye Worm". Eye pain and inflammation may occur. It does not cause blindness. Symptoms of brain inflammation, encephalitis, include headache and difficulty sleeping which may progress to coma and death. These symptoms are more likely to occur after treatment has been started and is presumed to be caused by a toxic reaction from killed microfilariae. Up to one third of those with *Loa loa* may have transient kidney and heart inflammation. Nerves and joints inflammation may develop from the immune system being activated and damaging these organs.

Diagnosis is through microscopic examination of microfilariae in a Giemsa-stained blood smear collected during the daytime. Blood samples at this time have a higher number of microfilariae that matches the daytime feeding pattern of the fly. It is also possible to identify adult worms migrating in the eye or passing through subcutaneous body tissue. Measuring antibodies may indicate that infection has occurred. If the IgM antibody is present this would indicate an ongoing infection. Positive IgG antibody may indicate a past infection. If both antibodies are positive, that would indicate an ongoing or recent infection. A PCR blood test is the most accurate test measuring *Loa loa* DNA.

If there is significant eye pain and discomfort or for diagnostic purposes surgery may be done to remove the worm from the eye. It would take a small cut and tweezers to physically remove the worm. Diethylcarbamazine is the treatment of choice and may be given at 8 to 10 mg/kg/day for three weeks. This would kill the adult worms and microfilariae. An alternative dosing schedule for Diethylcarbamazine would be on day one, a single oral dose of 1 mg/kg with a maximum dose of 50 mg; day 2, 1 mg/kg/dose, given three times a day with a maximum dose of 50 mg; day 3, 1 to 2 mg/kg per dose given three times a day and day 4 to day 21, 9 mg/kg/da divided into three doses.

About 50% are cured with a 21-day course of Diethylcarbamazine. Albendazole, Mebendazole and Ivermectin also have been used to kill the microfilariae. Ivermectin has no effect on adult worms. Those with a high microfilariae load when treated with Diethylcarbamazine or Albendazole may develop encephalitis. This may be the result of toxic products produced by microfilariae death and the body's own immune system response to those triggers. To reduce complications, give the medications in a lower dose over a longer period of time to minimize the occurrence of encephalitis or pretreat only with Albendazole. Treatment with Ivermectin seems to promote the microfilariae passing into the cerebrospinal fluid avoiding and escaping its effects. If after treatment any symptoms recur, then repeat a full course of therapy.

There is no vaccination for *Loa loa*. General preventive measures include wearing long pants and long sleeves. If there is a need to be outdoors during daytime fly feeding or indoors with no air conditioning or window screens. Effective insect repellent on exposed skin areas and washing clothes with a Permethrin based product will serve as additional protective measures. Travelers may receive prophylactic Diethylcarbamazine, a 300 mg dose once a week especially if they will have long-term exposure like peace corps volunteers or military deployment.

Amebic Dysentery.
Amebic Liver Abscess

Entamoeba histolytica

Entamoeba histolytica is found mainly in developing parts of the world with poor or limited water sanitation facilities. Estimates are that more than 1 billion people worldwide do not have access to safe food and clean drinking water. Because of this at-risk population there are 50 to 100 million cases of amebic disease worldwide causing as many as 100,000 deaths a year. Of these, 15,000 occur in children less than five years of age. In endemic areas 80 percent of all infants may be infected with *Entamoeba histolytica*.

Infection occurs through ingestion of food and water contaminated with *Entamoeba histolytica* cysts. Areas where contaminated infected human feces are used as a fertilizer increases the risk of infection. Ice cubes frozen from contaminated water have also been found to be another source for *Entamoeba histolytica* infection. There is a high rate of amebic infection in Mexico, Africa, India and parts of Central and South America. It is prevalent in developing countries in the world but may be seen anywhere because of international travel. Cases occurring in developed countries are a result of migrants and also travelers returning to their home from endemic areas.

Entamoeba cysts are resistant and may survive long periods in different environmental conditions. When they are ingested, they pass into the intestinal tract where in the terminal ileum, the last segment of the small intestines, cysts will release trophozoites. The trophozoites will pass into the large intestine (colon) where they multiply. Some trophozoites may penetrate the lining of the colon and ingest and kill the epithelial lining cells. From there they may pass to other organs particularly the liver, lung and brain. Some trophozoites with the favorable environment in the colon will develop into mature cysts and be passed in the feces. Both trophozoites and cysts may be seen in a stool sample. However, only the cysts are infectious. Trophozoites rapidly die in the environment and when ingested are killed by the gastric acids in the stomach.

Most infections are self-limited or asymptomatic. As many as 90% of those infected may become asymptomatic carriers, harboring *Entamoeba* but showing no symptoms or signs of illness. Carriers will pass infectious cysts in their stool, serving as a source for the spread of infection. As many as 4 to 10% of children carriers may progress and develop amebic diarrhea. Certain host genes seem to protect while others promote symptoms of illness to occur. The content of the intestinal flora also affects the degree of symptoms that develop. If or when symptoms occur, they may have a gradual onset over 3 to 4 weeks up to seven months after the onset of the infection.

Some infected individuals will develop symptoms of colitis/dysentery or liver abscess as soon as four days after cyst ingestion. Individuals who live in endemic areas may have chronic or repeated infections. Children may not be as ill as adults with *Entamoeba* infection. A child with *Entamoeba* infection may simply have diarrhea with no mucus or blood in their feces. However, it is possible for infection to be more severe and cause symptoms of "dysentery" with bloody or mucousy diarrhea, abdominal pain, cramping, fever and weight loss. As many as 15 to 33% of cases of *Entamoeba histolytica* diarrhea will be full blown dysentery.

With *Entamoeba histolytica* infection a child may have poor growth due to malnutrition. A mass of ameba may cause blockage in the large intestine interfering with fecal elimination. Trophozoites may spread to other organs, especially the liver producing an abscess. Infection of the heart and lungs occurs by extension from liver infection. There may be damage to blood vessels including thrombosis (blood clotting) of the hepatic vein and inferior vena cava. Large liver abscesses may produce mechanical compression of these blood vessels. Specific factors that promote disease spread to other organs have not been determined but may additionally be genetic or related to the individual's immune system function.

There may be as many as 50,000 deaths annually from amebic liver disease. Amebic liver disease is overall uncommon in children. The trophozoites pass from the large intestine lining through blood vessels back to the liver. Individuals who have an impaired immune system have an increased risk of amebic liver abscesses. For travelers, signs of a liver abscess may occur as soon as 2 to 4 weeks but more likely 8 to 20 weeks after return from an endemic area. For some individuals onset of symptoms may be delayed for years to decades.

Those with a liver abscess may have an enlarged tender liver however other symptoms may occur for months before the liver enlarges. They will have pain under the right rib margin that may go up the right chest to the shoulder. They may develop fever, sweating, cough, malaise, hiccoughs from diaphragm irritability, loss of appetite and weight loss. Fewer than 10 percent of those with a liver abscess will have jaundice and less than 1/3 will have diarrhea. Children with amebic liver abscess are less likely to have abdominal pain and more likely to have high fever and abdominal distention. Only 10 to 35% of those with a liver abscess will have gastrointestinal symptoms including abdominal cramping, nausea, vomiting, abdominal distention, diarrhea or constipation. Often they have a history of dysentery in the previous year.

As many as 10% of those with a liver abscess may have infection spread by either rupture of an abscess or spread of trophozoites through the blood and lymphatic system. Through these routes a liver abscess may spread disease to the abdomen causing peritonitis, chest causing lung and heart inflammation or abscesses or spread to the brain. Infection in the abdomen would cause a bloated, tender abdomen and fever. Symptoms of lung involvement are shortness of breath, chest pain, coughing and coughing up blood.

About 3% of those with a liver abscess may have infection extend into the sac around the heart, the pericardium. Symptoms of heart involvement would be severe chest pain, heart muscle inflammation either pericarditis or myocarditis, abscess formation in the heart and heart failure. Up to 4% of those with a liver abscess have trophozoites disseminate through the bloodstream to the brain. With brain infection there will be an abrupt onset of headache and seizures. If left untreated, brain infection will rapidly progress to death.

The gold standard for diagnosing *Entamoeba* is observing cysts or trophozoites in a stool sample. However, it is of limited value because its accuracy is limited by visually observing parasites in the stool which involves both skill and luck. Blood testing would show an elevated white blood cell count indicating inflammation or infection and elevated liver enzymes, alkaline phosphatase and transaminases indicating liver inflammation. The blood or stool PCR test is more accurate identifying *Entamoeba* DNA. Fecal PCR testing is 100 times more accurate than microscopy of a fecal sample. Stool studies are usually negative for those with a liver abscess. Those with a liver abscess do not routinely shed ameba in their feces. Serology tests measuring IgG antibody will show evidence of infection but not distinguish between it being recent or in the past. A positive IgM antibody titer is more consistent with an active ongoing or recent infection. In any case there may be a one-week delay from the beginning of the infection until the body makes enough antibody to produce a measurable positive serology test.

Imaging studies, x rays, ultrasound, computed tomography (CT), magnetic resonance imaging (MRI) will show abscesses if present. *Entamoeba* abscesses will have a round ring around the abscess when it is healing. There may be varying degrees of calcification noted. CT or ultrasound guided needle aspiration may provide infective fluid for microscopic analysis or PCR testing. Colonoscopy with biopsy of the infected terminal ileum or colon with microscopic examination will show invasive parasites and damage to the intestinal lining.

Previous infection will not prevent new infections from occurring. Infection may tend to recur despite appropriate treatment of previous infections. Additional infections may be milder or asymptomatic and seen in those living in endemic areas with frequent exposure to infective cysts. Large abscesses, those greater than 10 cm (almost 4 inches) in diameter may be drained to reduce the risk of rupture and spread to adjacent organs as well as to reduce the physical pressure on adjacent organs.

Aspiration of an abscess may be done for those not responding to treatment or for diagnostic consideration providing a sample for analysis. Needle aspiration does not improve treatment results. However, drainage with a catheter has been shown to be more effective in both draining fluid and producing faster clinical and radiological improvement.

Treatment does make a difference. The mortality rate for an uncomplicated liver abscess is less than 1% if treated early. Early evaluation of the liver through ultrasonography or computer tomography is critical. If treatment is delayed, the death rate may be as high as 17% especially if the abscess is large, there are multiple abscesses, or it has spread to the brain. Treat with specific agents to eliminate invasive disease, trophozoites have spread to different organs. Metronidazole is still the oral medicine of choice. It is dosed 30–50 mg/kg/day divided into 3 equal doses for 10 days. Other choices would be Tinidazole 50 mg/kg/day for 3 days, Secnidazole 30 mg/kg one time dose, Ornidazole 25 mg/kg/day for 5 to 10 days. After a course of any of these, up to 40 to 60% will still have parasites in their intestine. Agents that eliminate non-invasive disease, trophozoites and cysts that are in the intestines are Paromomycin given 25–30 mg/kg/day divided into 3 equal doses for 7 days, Diiodohydroxyquin 30–40 mg/kg/day divided into 3 equal doses for 20 days and Diloxanide 20 mg/kg/day divided into 3 equal doses for 10 days.

After the initial treatment with Metronidazole, a course of either Tinidazole, Secnidazole or Ornidazole should be routinely administered to produce a parasitological cure. It is recommended for those with an abscess and treatment failure or relapse, drain the abscess either by needle or preferably catheter placement and give a longer course of medication. Also give a longer course of medication for those with treatment failure for amebic dysentery. If there is a concern about secondary bacterial infection, then treat it with an oral antibiotic like Azithromycin or Clindamycin.

There is no effective vaccination for *Entamoeba histolytica*. For those living or visiting endemic areas, precautions are proper hygiene and appropriate elimination of infected material. Cook all foods thoroughly and before consumption wash each produce, vegetables and fruits with treated water. Avoid use of untreated water. Hygiene and hand washing are important components to staying healthy. Probiotics help to re-colonize the gastrointestinal tract and when given with Zinc promotes healing of the intestinal tract. Maintain appropriate hydration with Gatorade and if diarrhea is severe give it undiluted and avoid milk and dairy products.

Amebic Meningoencephalitis. Amebic Keratitis. Granulomatous Amebic Encephalopathy

Naegleria fowleri
Acanthamoeba species

Acanthamoeba and *Naegleria* are free living protozoans that may produce severe illness in people. They may commonly be found in the environment and produce disease in both healthy and immunocompromised children. Their diagnosis and treatment may be delayed. The response to treatment may be overall poorly tolerated, complicated and ineffective.

Naegleria fowleri

Naegleria fowleri is the cause of primary amebic meningoencephalitis. This is a rapidly progressive, fulminant, necrotizing, hemorrhagic, fatal brain infection that occurs in both healthy children and young adults. From this description it is obvious that it is a bad disorder. It exists in 3 stages, an invasive reproductive trophozoite, a non-feeding and nonreplicating form with two flagella, and a dormant resistant cyst.

The trophozoites are a free-living stage the live on bacteria and also divides in two. The trophozoite may proliferate in the warm summer months. If the environment begins to change unfavorably it will produce two flagella that allow it to be mobile and move effectively out of that area. This stage does not eat nor divide. It may revert into the trophozoite when environmental conditions are favorable. If environmental conditions become very unfavorable, it may transform into the resistant cyst stage.

This ameba enters the body through the nose and will penetrate the lining of the nose through the action of its own enzymes and the body's immune system response. It will pass along the olfactory nerve back into the brain. From the time that the parasite enters the nasal passageways until onset of illness may be 24 hours up to 5 to 7 days. This incubation period is the result of the individual's overall health status and numbers of parasites taken into the body during exposure. The more parasites taken in, the more rapid the onset of symptoms.

Infection causes pressure to build up in the brain. This results in sudden onset of a bad headache along the forehead and side of the head, then high fever, stiff neck, nausea, vomiting, altered taste or smell, and restlessness. This may be followed by light sensitivity, double vision, nosebleed, lethargy, bizarre behavior, confusion, seizures, shallow rapid breathing and coma. Death may occur within a week due to the increased brain pressure causing the brain to be pushed down or herniate into the spinal column.

Diagnosis is made by microscopic examination of biopsy brain tissue or spinal fluid showing the trophozoites. A Giemsa or Wright stain of the sample makes it easier to visualize trophozoites. Special staining procedures like immunofluorescence increases the accuracy of observation. Only the trophozoites grow and are seen in the brain biopsies. Cysts are not seen in the brain. A PCR test on spinal fluid or biopsy brain material may be positive showing Naegleria DNA.

Serology test may be negative because there is insufficient time to make measurable antibody. Conversely people who do not have primary amebic meningoencephalitis may have measurable antibodies from their previous exposure to non-or lesser pathogenic strains of *Naegleria*. These antibodies may have little or no protective value in preventing serious disease. These antibodies have been reported for individuals in New Zealand, California and the Southeastern United States. A measurable titer may also occur in those rare few who have recovered from primary amebic meningoencephalitis. Probably there are more cases occurring worldwide but go unreported due to delay in their diagnosis and their rapid progression to death.

No standard treatment has been developed for primary amebic meningoencephalitis. This is because most children die before any potentially effective medication may be started or have time to work. Typically, treatment is delayed because of uncertainty of their diagnosis with an incomplete history of water exposure and lack of awareness about the disease. Often, it is only diagnosed after death. Delay in treatment increases the likelihood the child will not survive.

Multiple combination treatments have been employed with most centering around Amphotericin B given over 10 days both intravenously 0.5 to 0.7 mg/kg/day combined with 25 to 300 µg dose given every 48 to 72 hours through a catheter into the brain or spinal column (intrathecal) because Amphotericin B does not pass from the bloodstream into the brain. This has been combined with Rifampin, Azithromycin, Miconazole and Ornidazole. All medications except Amphotericin B are dosed at 10 mg/kg/day for 28 days. Azithromycin has been shown to kill trophozoites. Miltefosine 50 mg twice a day has been combined with these medications. Other combinations that have been used are intravenous and intrathecal Amphotericin B and Miconazole with oral Rifampin. Another alternative combination is intravenous Dexamethasone dosed at 0.6 mg/kg/day in four divided doses for four days, Amphotericin B and Fluconazole with oral Rifampin. From these aggressive and combined therapies, it is obvious that treatment of primary amebic meningoencephalitis is a desperate undertaking.

There is no vaccination for prevention of *Naegleria fowleri* infections. Maintaining effective levels of chlorine is effective for swimming pools, Naegleria is killed by chlorine. At best, recreational water sources may be monitored for the presence of *Naegleria*. Otherwise, it is an individual's responsibility and accountability to avoid bathing, swimming or diving in warm freshwater (lakes, ponds, rivers and creeks). Do not immerse your head under water. If this is not possible to avoid, then use nasal plugs to prevent or minimize water in the nasal passageways. Nasal irrigation with the saline or Netty pot flush may remove likely area before it has a chance to become established.

Acanthamoeba

Amebic keratitis. Granulomatous Amebic Encephalopathy

Acanthamoeba has worldwide distribution, but most cases have been reported in the United States. It exists in two states, the trophozoite and resistant cyst. The trophozoite is the growing and dividing form. When environmental conditions become unfavorable it rounds up and forms a resistant cyst. When conditions are again favorable, it will become active and the trophozoite leaves the cyst. *Acanthamoeba* trophozoites and cysts are found in water, soil, and may be airborne recovered in air samples. Water samples include fresh and brackish water, waste sewage, rivers, seas, oceans, ocean sediments, rainwater, lakes, ponds, swimming pools, hot springs, tap and city water, fountains, mineral and bottled water, dust, potting soil, air conditioning units, cooling towers for electric and nuclear power plants, dental offices and dialysis clinics. They may be found on fresh vegetables, fruits and mushrooms, nasal swabs, throat swabs and infected ear drainage. It may spread through the nose, bloodstream and breaks in the skin. Infection may occur any time of the year.

Acanthamoeba infection is more likely to occur in children with immune system deficiencies, diabetes, autoimmune disorders, organ transplants, HIV/AIDS, disability, those chronically ill but also in healthy children. *Acanthamoeba* may harbor different types of *Mycobacterium* and *Legionella* that its trophozoites have ingested. Infection is dependent on the number of amebae taken in during the exposure to the contaminated source. The more ameba taken in, the more likely infection will occur and have disease progression. Additionally impaired status of the immune system and invasiveness of the specific *Acanthamoeba* strain affect onset of infection.

The onset of symptoms for Granulomatous Amebic Encephalitis is slow and insidious over several weeks to months. Symptoms of amebic encephalitis are altered mental status, disorientation, hallucinations, weakness and numbness of facial muscles, headache especially around the forehead, behavioral changes, irritability, altered taste and smell, neck stiffness, elevated or sub normal body temperature, seizures and coma.

Trophozoites excrete different enzymes that destroy host tissue that is then used for nutrition and also promotes spread to and destruction of the brain and other host tissues. The host immune response to *Acanthamoeba* may also produce additional tissue injury. The entire brain shows damage. Once the brain is involved and symptoms develop, death may occur in eight days up to several months. The mortality rate is 97 to 98% for chronic granulomatous amebic encephalitis. There will be areas of dead and hemorrhaged brain that may look like a tumor. *Acanthamoeba* cysts in the air may pass all the way through the bronchial tubes to the air exchange spaces, alveoli, and cause pneumonia. Specific lung changes are seen on a chest x-ray. Ameba may be recovered from lung/bronchial washings. Those with immunosuppression may also have ulcerative skin lesions on the chest and extremities.

Acanthamoeba may get into the eye and produce inflammation, infection and damage, keratitis. It may be in contaminated contact lense solutions especially those homemade. It may involve only one eye. It may occur because of eye injury and is more likely to occur in contact lense wearers. Estimates are 85 to 88% of all cases of *Acanthamoeba* keratitis occur and those wearing contact lenses. *Acanthamoeba* may produce ulceration and deep tissue damage of the cornea causing severe eye pain, light sensitivity, decreased visual acuity and blindness if not treated promptly and effectively.

It is difficult to diagnose, and most cases are misidentified as bacterial, viral or fungal infections. Diagnosis is initially based on a strong clinical suspicion and confirmed through laboratory testing. Microscopic examination and PCR of biopsied skin or brain material are tools that aid in the diagnosis. Both trophozoites and cysts are found in biopsies of infected brain material but not in spinal fluid. Cultures of biopsied material may grow ameba trophozoites. Serology blood test would show evidence of exposure to *Acanthamoeba* but unless showing IgM antibody would not indicate an ongoing infection and illness. Detection of antibodies may be from environmental exposure to non-or lesser pathogenic strains of *Acanthamoeba*. There is no simple solution for treatment of *Acanthamoeba* disease. The cyst stage is resistant to antibiotics and amoebicidal agents. Once cysts release trophozoites, they are the target for treatment. Various combinations of medications have been used to treat *Acanthamoeba* illness. *Acanthamoeba* may be successfully treated if it has not spread to the brain. Before discontinuing therapy, the child should be rescreened with cultures, PCR, biopsied material if accessible to confirm they no longer have active disease.

For Granulomatous Amebic Encephalitis:
Miltefosine as a single agent or add 1 or more of the following
Fluconazole plus Sulfadiazine plus Pyrimethamine.
Trimethoprim-Sulfamethoxazole plus Rifampin plus Ketoconazole.
Treat for 4 to 6 months.

For *Acanthamoeba* Keratitis:
The most effective agent is Polyhexamethylene Biguanide eyedrops with or without Brolene eyedrops.
Keratoplasty is done to remove any residual scar tissue after the infection has been effectively treated and all medicine has been completed.
Treat for 6 months up to 1 year.

For *Acanthamoeba* Respiratory Infection/Pneumonia:
Amphotericin B with one of the following in combination: Trimethoprim or miltefosine or Voriconazole or Pentamidine or Fluorocytosine or Itraconazole.
Treat for 4 to 6 months.

For Cutaneous *Acanthamoeba*:
Topical Chlorhexidine and Ketoconazole.
Treat for 4 to 6 months.

Preventive measures are more reliant on surveillance for *Acanthamoeba* in environmental sources and good common sense to avoid contact and situations that may lead to *Acanthamoeba* exposure and infection. The cyst stage is resistant to chlorine. Surveillance and culturing of recreational exposures is an important component protecting individuals from *Acanthamoeba*. This is especially important for anyone who is immunosuppressed or immunocompromised. Avoid submersion in potentially contaminated waters.

Proper care of contact lenses is critical to prevent *Acanthamoeba* keratitis. Wash hands with soap and water before touching contact lenses. Wear and replace contact lenses as recommended by the manufacturer and your eye care specialist. Maintain storage and cleaning as recommended by the manufacturer and healthcare provider. Remove contact lenses before water activities including hot tubs, swimming and bathing. Keep regular eye checkups.

Disinfecting the skin with bleach water soaks after recreational water activities will reduce the chances of ulcerative skin sores. However, it has no effect on the ameba that have entered the nasal passageways. Flushing the nasal passageways with a Neti pot or saline rinse may help to irrigate and remove cysts and trophozoites in the sinuses and nasal passageways.

Ascaris lumbricoides

Roundworm/Nematode

Ascaris lumbricoides is the most common helminth (parasitic worm) infection producing chronic infection in more than 800 million people worldwide. It is one of several soil transmitted helminths. *Ascaris* survives and is transmitted year around in subtropical and tropical areas of Asia, Sub-Saharan Africa and the Americas. In other more hostile climactic areas, the eggs are viable in the soil for months and transmitted during certain favorable seasons of the year. It may infect children of all ages with increasing intensity from infancy through preschool and school-age children. Children 5 to 15 years of age have the highest load of *Ascaris* due to their environmental exposures. *Ascaris* has different larval stages that mature and migrate through the body.

Adult *Ascaris* worms live in the human intestinal tract. They have a thick surface called a cuticle that makes it resistant to digestive enzymes. An adult worm may grow and survive in the intestinal tract for one up to two years. An adult female *Ascaris* may produce and release up to 200,000 eggs a day that pass in the stool. These eggs are very resistant and may survive in the environment for two months without soil and up to 15 years in favorable soil and environmental conditions. The eggs are not immediately infectious and depending on the environmental temperature may take 10 to 50 days to embryonate and become infectious in the soil. Old, not fresh feces would be contagious.

A new infection occurs when the eggs are orally ingested, hatch in response to bile acids and develop into stage 2 larvae in the small intestine. The stage 2 larvae burrow into the intestinal wall and are carried by the blood vessels to the liver. There they pass through the blood to the lung tissue where they develop into stage 3 larvae. These larvae will then travel up and out of the bronchial tubes into the epiglottis and then are swallowed back into the stomach. They will pass for a second time into the small intestines and continue development into the adult worms. This migration process may take 2 to 3 months. Migration of the larvae will activate the host immune system resulting in high levels of eosinophils in the bloodstream and elevated IgE antibody levels. These eosinophils may also lodge in tissues and organs that are inflamed from larvae migration.

Most infections will have no symptoms. However, when symptoms occur, they will vary depending upon the number and different stages of larvae migrating through the body and finally becoming established in the intestinal tract. The greater the number, the greater the symptoms. During the migratory or "visceral stages", there may be abdominal pain, nausea, and vomiting as the larvae pass through the intestines and liver. When larvae pass into the lungs, there may be shortness of breath, wheezing, spasms of the bronchial tubes with asthma-like symptoms and eosinophils infiltrating the lungs.

Adult worms in the intestinal tract produce a chronic infection causing abdominal distention, nausea and pain. Additional complications from malabsorption are deficiencies of vitamin A, fat and Iodine, protein loss, weight loss, impaired growth with slowed mental and developmental delay.

Humans and pigs are very similar in their physiology. The pig roundworm *Ascaris suum* may also cause human disease. Many pig farms even in the United States will have infected pigs. Anyone exposed to infected pigs, pig manure or soil contaminated with infected pig feces is at risk to ingest their eggs. This will result in similar symptoms and pass through the same stages as the human roundworm.

The adult female may weigh 4 up to 9 grams (0.009–0.02 pounds) and be as long as 12–15.5 inches. The male worms may weigh 2 to 3 grams (0.005–0.007 pounds) and be 6 to 12 inches long. They are more commonly found in the jejunum segment of the small intestines and feed on intestinal contents. In heavy infections they may be found competing for space anywhere in the gastrointestinal tract.

Children may have a greater number of adult worms due to repeated exposure and ingestion. Because of the large size of the adult *Ascaris* worms and small size of the terminal ileum, the last portion of the small intestines, bowel obstruction may occur requiring surgical removal. Other acute emergency bowel changes from *Ascaris* infection may be twisting or telescoping of the bowels, perforation of the intestinal wall and infection in the abdominal cavity (peritonitis). The corresponding high levels of IgE antibody or acute lung damage from larval migration may cause spasm of the bronchial tubes and wheezing. These are asthma-like symptoms but not asthma.

The adult worms may move from the intestines into the appendix, gall bladder, liver, bile and pancreatic ducts and stomach into the back of the throat. These migrating worms may lead to appendicitis, inflamed liver, gallbladder and pancreas respectively. They may be found in the nose and eustachian tubes. Dead worms are carried out of the gastrointestinal tract in feces. If they are in the bile duct, they may cause gallstone formation. If surgery is needed, either to remove worms or repair damaged organs, it may be done endoscopically or if the damage is extensive, may require "open" surgery.

Diagnosis is made by identifying adult *Ascaris* worms or eggs seen microscopically in the stool. The adult worms may be seen in the feces without a microscope. There may be variation in the rate of egg excretion, and it is possible to examine a bucket of stool and miss seeing worms or eggs. The number of eggs in the stool has no correlation to the number of adults in the host. However, a low number of worms may also decrease egg recovery.

Methods that increase the concentration of eggs in the stool will increase recovery and positive results. Alternatively, a polymerase chain reaction (PCR) test measuring *Ascaris* DNA may be used to accurately detect fewer numbers of eggs and show ongoing infection with more than one type of soil transmitted parasite.

There is no effective *Ascaris* vaccination for people or pigs. Treat all infected individuals including those both symptomatic and asymptomatic with oral Benzimidazole either 400 mg of Albendazole or 500 mg of Mebendazole. Cure rates with a single dose are 88 and 95% respectively. Rapid reinfection occurs making it less likely mass elimination is possible. Deworming specific populations is effective in reducing the numbers of *Ascaris* but this is not sustainable. However, it may be worthwhile in endemic areas to deworm individuals every six months who are exposed to pigs. Only improvement in sanitation with proper disposal of human and animal feces, access to clean water and improved hygiene will reduce community transmission and reinfection with *Ascaris*.

Babesia

Babesiosis
Babesia microti
Babesia divergens
Babesia WA 1

Babesiosis is an illness caused by a parasite of the species *Babesia* that infects and survives inside the host's red blood cells (intraerythrocytic). There are more than 100 different species that may infect animals and mammals, with three predominant types affecting humans, *Babesia microti, Babesia divergens* and *Babesia* WA1. There is a worldwide distribution limited by the habitat of the *Ixodes* tick which is responsible for spreading this parasite through blood feeding. This is a small tick the size of a poppyseed. The range for these ticks has been increasing over the past 20 years.

Babesia cases have been reported in Germany, France, Denmark, Norway, the Netherlands, mainland and Northwestern China, Egypt, India, Japan, Australia, South Africa, Democratic Republic of the Congo, rural Bolivia, Northwestern Columbia and the United States. Worldwide sporadic cases have been reported in Mexico, Mozambique, Taiwan, the Canary Islands, the Ivory Coast and the Sudan.

There are around 2000 cases reported in the United States each year. This is an underestimation of the actual number because most cases are asymptomatic or have mild symptoms and go undiagnosed. In the United States it occurs in endemic areas including the Northeastern and upper Midwestern states, Connecticut, Delaware, Maine, Maryland, Minnesota, Vermont, Virginia, New Hampshire, New Jersey, Washington DC, Wisconsin, New York, and Pennsylvania. It is highly endemic from New Jersey to Cape Cod and Eastern Long Island, Shelter Island, Nantucket and Martha's Vineyard. Sporadic cases have been reported in Missouri, Kentucky, Arkansas, Washington state, California and Michigan.

Cases have occurred in animals since biblical times producing plague in cattle during the time of Rameses II. It was shown in 1891 to be the cause of Texas cattle fever. In 1896, ticks were identified as the source for this illness. The first reported case in humans was in 1957 in Yugoslavia and the first human case in the United States was in California in 1966. Those at risk of developing Babesiosis spend a lot of time outside or have contact with livestock. Specific groups at risk are hikers, campers, gardeners, yard workers, park rangers, forest workers and farmers. Individuals who have had their spleen removed, have received an organ transplant, the elderly, newborn premature infants, those who have an illness or are on medicines that suppress their immune system or have immune system deficiencies are also at risk for both *Babesia* illness and to have more severe disease.

Babesia is spread by an *Ixodes* tick feeding on infected animal reservoirs. There are a number of animal reservoirs including the white footed mouse, raccoons, foxes, skunks, wolves, cattle, horses, sheep, goats, pigs, dogs and cats. The tick takes in the gametocyte parasite stage. This stage does not occur in humans. In the tick gut gametocytes fuse to produce the ookinete stage. This stage will penetrate the gut lining of the tick and pass to the salivary gland. There it continues development and forms sporozoites. It may form as many as 100,000 sporozoites that are infectious for humans and animal reservoirs. The sporozoites are introduced through tick feeding into the bloodstream and attach and penetrate red blood cells. In red blood cells the sporozoites mature into the trophozoites. Trophozoites continue to develop and bud to form the next stage, the merozoite. Inside the red blood cells, the merozoites remain close together and look like a Maltese cross.

In the animal reservoirs a small number of merozoites will develop into gametes. Infected red blood cells rupture releasing the merozoites. They may in turn attach to and penetrate additional red blood cells. This process may continue producing lysis of a significant number of red blood cells leading to severe anemia. There is no human-to-human spread by tick feeding. The gamete stage only develops in reservoir animals and must go through an intermediate animal host to complete its complex life cycle.

It may take 36 to 54 hours of tick feeding to transfer the parasite. Alternatively, it may be transmitted by blood transfusions that are contaminated with *Babesia*. The estimates are that out of every 1 million donated units of blood, six will be contaminated with *Babesia*. However, blood collected in endemic areas carries a much higher rate of *Babesia* contamination. In Rhode Island, an endemic area for *Babesia*, 1/21,000 blood units are contaminated with *Babesia*.

There is no testing done to screen donated blood for *Babesia*. The donor is screened only through a questionnaire determining if they are at high risk of acquired *Babesia*. Symptoms may develop one to six weeks after a contaminated transfusion with an average incubation period of 36 days. Newborns may acquire *Babesia* from their infected mothers if infected or if ill from a contaminated blood transfusion.

It is estimated that 25% of all cases of *Babesia* in adults and 50% of all infections in children will be asymptomatic or have mild disease. For this reason, it is underrecognized or due to just a simple lack of awareness of this illness by healthcare providers. It has a similar distribution to Lyme disease and 2 up to 66% of those with *Babesia* infection are co-infected with Lyme. There is a clustering of cases with more than 70% of those ill with *Babesia* having symptoms occur in the spring and summer between June and the beginning of September.

Babesiosis will produce an unexplained flu-like illness with hemolytic anemia and a low platelet count. Symptoms are the combined result of direct damage to the red blood cells from the parasite and activated elevated levels of components of the immune system that produce tissue and organ damage. The most common symptoms are fever, chills, headache, fatigue, joint and bone pain, and muscle pain that may develop 1 to 6 weeks after an infected tick bite. These symptoms occur in mild to moderate illness and are correlated with parasitemia of less than 4%.

Individuals who are at high risk for severe disease have a more difficult time course and more severe disease. They will have a low platelet count (the body's clotting cells). Due to accelerated lysis/rupture of the red blood cells they will have more severe anemia leading to kidney, lung, heart distress and failure. For those with severe disease and severe enough to require hospitalization, especially the elderly and those with no spleen, they have a fatality rate of 2 to 9%.

The diagnosis of *Babesia* is through identification of the parasite in stained thin blood smears microscopically visualized by a technician. Either a Giemsa or Wright stain are the stains of choice. However, the accuracy is limited by the number of red blood cells that are infected by *Babesia*. If the infection rate is less than 0.1%, there may be an insufficient number of infected red blood cells to microscopically find the parasite.

Unfortunately, *Babesia* may be microscopically confused for malaria, and it is also possible for an individual to be simultaneously co-infected with both malaria and *Babesia*. There are tests that measure IgG and IgM antibodies the body produces in response to the infection. The presence of IgG *Babesia* antibodies shows that at some point the parasite was in the body but does not confirm active or on-going infection. The presence of IgM antibodies would suggest a more recent or on-going infection.

The immunofluorescent test (IFAT) will identify Babesia but is not specific to identify the causative species. All serology tests may be negative in the early stages of the infection. There are other more sensitive and accurate molecular tests that may be performed, a polymerase chain reaction test (PCR) or nucleic acid amplification test (NAT, NAAT). The PCR is 2 to 100 times more sensitive than diagnosing *Babesia* from microscopic examination of a blood smear. Molecular tests are more specific and may measure species specific DNA of both dead and living forms.

Successful treatments have been developed and refined over the years. One recommendation is to only treat individuals who have active disease and are symptomatic regardless of their serology or PCR tests results. For those with mild to moderate disease, oral medications are used. For severe disease, those with parasitemia of greater than 10% or a high-risk group for complications, start with oral medication. They may eventually require intravenous medication. A combination of Azithromycin and Atovaquone are recommended for treatment of Babesiosis. For those with more severe disease, severe anemia, impairment of kidney, lungs or heart function, a combination of Clindamycin and Quinine is given.

The combination of Azithromycin and Atovaquone may have fewer adverse side effects. The recommended length of treatment with either of these combinations is seven days but may be extended for longer periods up to 28 days depending upon their clinical response and improvement. An improved platelet count, the body's clotting cells, may be the first indicator of improvement.

For adults, Clindamycin is given 20–40 mg/kg/day divided into 3 equal doses of 300 to 600 mg intravenously over 6 hours or maximum of 600 mg given orally every 8 hours. This is combined with Quinine 25 mg/kg/day divided into 3 equal oral doses with a maximum for each dose of 650 mg given every 6 to 8 hours. An alternative for adults would be Azithromycin 500 to 1000 mg given on day 1 and 200–250 mg is given on days 2 through 5. This is combined with Atovaquone 750 mg given every 12 hours.

This combination is used for those with more serious disease and those requiring hospitalization.

Children are dosed based on their body weight. Clindamycin is given 7–10 mg/kg oral or intravenously in 3 equal doses over 6 to 8 hours with a maximum dose of 600 mg per dose. Quinine is orally dosed at 8 mg/kg every eight hours with a maximum dose of 650 mg per dose. This combination is preferred for pediatric patients. For Azithromycin, children receive 10 mg/kg on the first day dose, maximum dose 500 mg. Dose on day 2 through 5 is 5 mg/kg per dose with a maximum dose of 250 mg. The recommended oral dose of Atovaquone for children is 20 mg/kg every 12 hours with a maximum dose of 750 mg. Estimates are that 11% of all 10 to 19-year-olds and 73% of those 80 years of age and older will require hospitalization for more serious illness. Unfortunately, the mortality, death rate for hospitalized patients is 5 to 10%.

Those severely ill requiring hospitalization may receive a partial blood exchange removing some of their infected red blood cells and replacing it with uninfected blood. Babies, including premature babies and those severely ill from contaminated blood transfusions or acquiring the infection from their mother may receive a double volume exchange transfusion. Exchange transfusions may reduce the parasite load, parasitemia, by 50 to 90%. It also decreases the level of circulating immune system inflammatory products that continue to drive the body's autoimmune reaction.

Exchange transfusion, taking out infected blood and replacing it with donor blood, is recommended if an infected individual is having organ impairment or failure, severe anemia due to lysis of infected red blood cells or for any *Babesia* infection with more than 10% of their red blood cells infected. It may take three months after treatment for symptoms to resolve. For some there may be a persistent parasitemia even after effective treatment. The body will achieve a certain balance limiting the expansion of the number of infected red blood cells but not completely eradicating the illness. A recommendation is that if 3 months after treatment has been completed there is still a positive PCR, then retreat the individual.

The key for preventing babesiosis is to be smart about the environmental exposure risks and take all measures to limit tick exposure by as much as possible avoiding tick infested areas. Wearing light clothing, especially white, makes it easier to see ticks on clothing. It has been reported that dark clothing is less likely to attract ticks, but it may be just harder to see ticks on the dark clothing. Wear long sleeves, long pants, button collars, tuck pants into socks in shoes. Apply a product with DEET to exposed skin areas and to the edges of clothing.

Clothing may be washed in a Permethrin based laundry product which repels ticks and may be effective for 4 to 5 washings. If a tick has embedded in the skin, use fine tipped tweezers and grab the tick as close as possible to the skin level, not the body. Putting pressure or squeezing the tick body may cause more parasites to be pushed into the person. Environmental control of ticks through spraying programs may be overall ineffective and create toxic environmental conditions. Logistically it is not feasible or practical to try to remove or reduce the animal carrier reservoir population in each area or region.

Brain Cysts. Cysticercosis. Neurocysticercosis

Taenia solium

Cysticercosis and neurocysticercosis have been reported from every continent. However, those residing or traveling to areas of high occurrence for *Taenia solium* (pig tapeworm) infections have a higher risk of acquiring their eggs and developing infection. Estimates are that millions of people are infected worldwide. People may become infected with *Taenia solium* by ingesting eggs on fomites, food or water that has been contaminated with animal feces. Alternatively, people may ingest eggs of *Taenia solium* from poor hygiene, poor hand washing and autoinfection. As many as 15% of those with *Taenia* brain infection, neurocysticercosis also have intestinal *Taenia solium* infection and are the source of their own infection. It occurs in Mexico, Central America, Latin America, South America, Southeast Asia, Africa, China, India and Nepal.

Infection may involve any tissue in the body, skeletal muscle, brain, eyes, heart, lung, liver, abdomen and subcutaneous tissue. It is more serious when the infection is in the brain, nervous system and heart. When infection is in the brain it is called neurocysticercosis. Overall estimates are 2% of all those with *Taenia solium* infection also have neurocysticercosis. It more often occurs in Latin America and Asia. The prevalence of neurocysticercosis is estimated to be 1.2% in Brazil, 5.4% in Peru, 4.1% in Zambia and 7.4% in Rwanda. In certain areas of Guatemala, Mexico, Ecuador and Honduras up to 20% may have a positive test for *Taenia solium*. Neurocysticercosis may account for as many as 50,000 deaths per year.

Ingested eggs are digested in the stomach releasing the oncosphere. It will penetrate the intestinal wall and travel to different sites through the bloodstream. In about three months after infection started the oncosphere will produce a protective wall making a cyst called a coenuri. The cyst produces and secretes substances that block the body's own immune response. In time these protective substances become less effective, and the body's immune system will degenerate the cysts. There may be no symptoms until the cyst dies. This would trigger an immune system response producing inflammation. The severity of symptoms is directly related to the number of cysts present and their location in the body. Compared to adults, children are less likely to become infected and those who become infected are less likely to develop symptoms.

When cysts in the brain die, cerebritis or meningitis may develop. Initially there may be no symptoms of a brain infection. Nervous system symptoms may occur any time between 3 to 5 years after infection started or conversely be delayed up to 30 years. Initial symptoms may mimic a brain tumor. Migraine-like headaches, nausea, stiff neck and seizures may occur. As many as 50 to 70% of all those with neurocysticercosis will have recurring seizures. Up to 30% of epilepsy in underdeveloped countries is due to neurocysticercosis. Cysts in the brain may cause obstruction of cerebrospinal fluid flow resulting in swelling and inflammation of the brain. Four to 12% of those with neurocysticercosis will also have a stroke.

Other organs may be involved and produce varying symptoms. Cysts may occur in the eye producing double vision, bulging of the eyeball, eye pain, and vision loss. There may be blurry vision and retinal detachment. If cysts occur in muscles, they may produce a lump under the skin that may be tender. Cysts may occur in the heart producing heart rhythm abnormalities, heart weakness and failure. Cysts outside the heart or brain are less likely to produce symptoms.

There may be a delay from the beginning of the illness until the diagnosis is made. Evaluation would not be started until symptoms develop. Then a CT or MRI scan would identify the cyst and its location. This could be followed by fine needle aspiration with microscopic examination of the cystic material. PCR may also be run on material from this biopsy confirming *Taenia* DNA. Blood serology test may show positive IgG and/or IgM antibody for *Taenia solium*. Pediatric patients are more likely to have an increased number of blood eosinophils. For those with ocular cysticercosis, cysts may be seen in the eye.

Initially there may be mismanagement due to a delay in establishing the correct diagnosis. When treatment is started Albendazole is the medicine of choice. It is given 10–15 mg/kg/day divided into two equal doses for 10 to 14 days. It is taken with a fatty meal. Treatment may be extended up to 28 days. Single therapy with Albendazole produces a 68 to 70% cure rate. Praziquantel may be added on for additional benefit. When brain inflammation has occurred, individuals should also be treated with corticosteroids, 6–8 mg/kg/day divided into three equal daily doses given for 28 days. Then slowly taper the corticosteroid over the next 2 to 8 weeks. These medicines are not effective for cysts that have calcified. Cysts outside the central nervous system may be accessible for surgery. Up to one third of all those with neurocysticercosis will also have seizures. Control seizures with seizure medication. Unfortunately, there is no evidence that treating an asymptomatic child with cysticercosis or neurocysticercosis reduces their future development of neurologic symptoms.

There is a swine vaccination available for *Taenia solium*. This may be given to commercially raised pigs. Feral and home-grown swine in underdeveloped countries are not routinely vaccinated and remain an important unaddressed reservoir. Preventive measures are aimed at stopping egg ingestion. Proper cooking and preparation of vegetables and meat is critical. Wash cutting boards, counters, dishes and utensils with clean water. Don't drink untreated water. Travelers should drink bottled water or water that has been boiled. Health education, sanitation and proper hygiene when applied are also effective in reducing the occurrence of cysticercosis and neurocysticercosis.

Broad Fish Tapeworm

Diphyllobothrium latum
Diphyllobothrium pacificum
Diphyllobothrium nihonkaiense

Diphyllobothrium is a tapeworm with worldwide distribution. It is reported essentially in every continent except Antarctica. There are reports of cases from Taiwan, Korea, China, Japan, Finland, France, Switzerland, Italy, Russia, Siberia, New Zealand, Alaska, the Great Lakes of North America, Canada, the Pacific coast of South America, Peru and Chile. It will occur naturally or be brought in from endemic areas by travelers, immigrants and refugees or by imported infected fish. It is estimated that as many as 20 million people may be infected worldwide with the occurrence as high as 2% in coastal areas. The true occurrence is unknown because most infections remain asymptomatic.

There are multiple species of *Diphyllobothrium* but there are three major types infecting people matching up with specific geographic areas. *Diphyllobothrium latum* occurs in freshwater fish, pikes, trout, salmon, perch and mullets in Europe and North America. *Diphyllobothrium pacificum* occurs along the Pacific coast of South America and Asia and is found in marine fish, especially the Pacific salmon. *Diphyllobothrium nihonkaiense* occurs in the northern Pacific regions including Japan and North America. It likewise is spread through the Pacific salmon fish. It has also shown up as imported cases through infected fish throughout Europe and France. The occurrence of imported cases is on the rise because of the increasing popularity of eating raw, smoked or pickled freshwater fish, sushi, sashimi, gefilte fish, carpaccio and ceviche.

All kinds of animals including mammals, birds and reptiles may become infected by ingesting infected fish with the plerocercoid larvae. A wide range of mammals across the board including people, dogs, cats, bears, seals, minks, foxes and wolves may serve as a host for the broad fish tapeworm. Infection in these animals may serve as a source to keep returning broad fish tapeworm eggs to the environment and continuing infections. When an infected fish is ingested, the plerocercoid larva will excyst in the intestinal tract and over the next 2 to 6 weeks mature into an adult. An individual host may have single or multiple worms present at the same time. Adult worms may live for more than 30 years. An adult worm may produce 1 million eggs a day.

The unembryonated eggs will pass with feces into the water. In the water, eggs are stimulated to become embryonated (fertile) and transform into ciliated embryos. This stage will infect microcrustaceans, water fleas and copepods. In microcrustaceans, it develops into the procercoid larva. When a fish ingests the procercoid larva infected microcrustaceans, the procercoid larva will then migrate to the fish's muscle. There it develops into the plerocercoid larva and encysts. This is the infectious stage and is just waiting for the fish to be ingested by the next host. When this infected fish is ingested by an animal, the plerocercoid larva will excyst in the intestinal tract, usually the ileum and develop into an adult. The adults will produce and release eggs into the environment which continues the lifecycle.

Most children and adults with *Diphyllobothrium* have no symptoms. Those with a heavy worm load may have abdominal pain, bloating, nausea, vomiting, indigestion, diarrhea or constipation. They may have salt craving. Large or multiple worms could cause an intestinal obstruction, especially *Diphyllobothrium latum* which may be as long as 30 meters (nearly 100 feet). The *pacificum* and *nihonkaiense* species are smaller and these adults may reach 3 to 4 meters (10 to 13 feet) in length.

The adult worm will compete and take B12 from the host's intestines. It may render the person B12 and possibly folate deficient. This could produce a type of anemia called megaloblastic anemia causing weakness, loss of appetite, weight loss, dizziness and headache as well as neurological changes. Neurological changes would be tingling and numbness of the hands and feet, declining vision, balance and walking problems, loss of memory and mental alertness. Megaloblastic anemia is more likely to occur with a high number of worms at one time that have been present for 3 to 4 years.

Diagnosis of a *Diphyllobothrium* infection first requires a high index of suspicion in a symptomatic individual with a history of ingestion of raw, smoked, pickled, undercooked or imported fish. The diagnosis may be made by observing with microscopic examination of feces either *Diphyllobothrium* eggs or detached segments of the tapeworm called proglottids. PCR analysis of the feces would show *Diphyllobothrium* DNA. Worms may also be visualized and collected during colonoscopy.

Estimates are that 25 to 30% of all *Diphyllobothrium* infections will clear spontaneously without treatment. For those symptomatic and needing treatment, they would receive a single 15 up to 25 mg/kg dose of Praziquantel. A single treatment results in 100% cure. If B12 deficiency has developed, the individual would receive either oral or injections of B12 supplement. The feces should be rescreened for eggs or proglottids two months after treatment with Praziquantel.

There is no effective vaccination for *Diphyllobothrium*. The key to prevention is through education, how the worm is acquired, maintenance of proper sanitation measures and appropriate preparation to inactivate the plerocercoid larvae. Proper preparation of fish would be to first of all not eat raw, smoked, pickled or undercooked fish or fish imported from endemic areas of the world. If people insist on eating raw, smoked, pickled, undercooked or imported fish, then measures may be taken to inactivate the plerocercoid larvae. The fish may be made safe for consumption by deep freezing the fish at −10°C (14 F) for 24 to 48 hours, freeze and store the fish at −20°C (−4 F) for seven days, freeze the fish at −35°C (−31 F) for 15 hours, brine treat the fish with 12% sodium chloride, or cook the fish at 54 to 56°C (129 to 133 F) for five minutes.

Chagas Disease.
Sleeping Sickness

Trypanosoma
Trypanosomiasis
American Trypanosomiasis: Chagas disease.
  Trypanosoma cruzi
African Trypanosomiasis: Sleeping sickness.
  Trypanosoma brucei

Trypanosomes have a complex lifecycle requiring a specific intermediate vector host for its transmission of this illness. The vector is specific for the geographical area. In the Americas it is the kissing bug or cone nose bug and in African it is the tsetse fly. The pattern of illness is unique for each type of trypanosomiasis. Infection is limited to the endemic areas. However, with international travel, military personnel on assignment, immigrants and potential transfer by blood transfusions and organ transplants it will be diagnosed in non-endemic areas. This is a result of individuals infected in endemic areas leaving that area or returning home before becoming symptomatic.

There may be a delayed latency period between acquisition of the illness and onset of symptoms. Illness is always worse in any individual who has an immune system deficiency or is on medicines or has an illness that suppresses their immune system function. An alteration in their immune system function may reactivate chagas disease. Chagas disease may also cause congenital infections. Anyone spending time living or through travel in an endemic area should take all the necessary precautions, using an insect repellant, avoiding time outdoors when the insect vectors are feeding, use bed nets and avoid sleeping in dilapidated buildings. Keep insects out of food and beverages which are another potential source for infection.

Chagas disease, American Trypanosomiasis

Chagas disease is caused by the parasitic protozoan *Trypanosoma cruzi*. It will occur in endemic areas, Bolivia, Venezuela, Colombia, Central America, Mexico, the United States, Switzerland, Sweden and Spain. Cases in the United States have been reported in Southern and Western states, Texas, California, Tennessee and Louisiana. The kissing bug has been found in Delaware but there have been no reported cases. In the United States it is the hunters who are at the greatest risk to become infected with *Trypanosoma cruzi* from infected insects or contact with the infected blood or tissue of a gutted animals. It has been eradicated from Brazil, Chile, Paraguay and Uruguay. It is estimated that around 5.7 million people in Latin America and 9 million people worldwide are infected with *Trypanosoma cruzi*.

Each year there are around 56,000 new cases of chagas disease with approximately 12,000 deaths. As many as 240,000 people in the United States are infected with *Trypanosoma cruzi*. Individuals living in endemic areas are at a greater risk of acquiring this illness. In areas of the United States, hunters are at a higher risk for the disease because of outdoor activities increasing their exposure to the vector. They also have exposure from contaminated blood of infected reservoirs that have been killed and dressing carcasses. Initial stages of the illness are generally asymptomatic, a time when treatment is most effective. Heart disease onset may be delayed sometimes up to decades. However, when it begins, it is progressive and as many as 30% have worsening heart damage.

It is spread by the kissing bug or cone nose bug. They may live in nooks and crannies of buildings. This insect is found extending from Southern Argentina to the Southern half of the United States. It characteristically feeds at night. It has a complex life cycle involving different stages of development in different hosts. When the infected bug takes a blood meal, it defecates depositing infectious parasites (trypomastigotes) onto the skin. These parasites may enter breaks in the skin or be rubbed into the eyes. It may also be transmitted orally by food or drink contaminated with infected kissing bugs or their feces. The bug becomes infected by feeding on an infected person or infected animal. The animal reservoirs are limited to non-human mammalian hosts, and to be infectious would have the trypomastigotes in their bloodstream. For *Trypanosoma cruzi*, humans are not needed to complete the parasite lifecycle.

The trypomastigotes will pass into the insect midgut and multiplying. There they develop into the epimastigote stage. The epimastigote stage passes into the insect hindgut and develops into the infective trypomastigote stage. When transmitted to a mammalian host, the trypomastigote will pass into host cells and transform into the amastigote. When in the host cell, the amastigote will multiply and differentiate into the trypomastigote. As the host cell fills with trypomastigotes it will rupture releasing the trypomastigotes. They will spread to adjacent host cells or travel through the blood stream or lymphatic system. Their preferred host cells are muscle cells, especially the heart.

Infection occurs in endemic areas but may not be detected until those that are infected, travelers, immigrants or military personnel have returned to their non-endemic resident areas. Contaminated blood transfusions and organ transplants are additional ways it may be spread. Blood donors may only be screened through questionnaires and have a specified delay after returning from international travel.

Individuals at any age may become infected and develop acute disease the first time they are infected with *Trypanosoma cruzi*. They will develop nonspecific, usually mild signs a week or so after the parasite enters the body. Chagas disease may begin as an inflammatory skin sore called a chagoma that develops at the site of the parasite's entry into the body. This may be a red, swollen, firm area. The lymph nodes may also be swollen throughout the body. There may be fever, swelling of the face with painless swelling of the eyes, loss of appetite, malaise and just feeling bad. The liver and spleen may enlarge and be tender. If left untreated, symptoms gradually resolve over weeks to months and the individual becomes asymptomatic. However, it will invade subcutaneous tissue and muscle cells. Muscle cells, especially those in the heart, are a preferred site for cell invasion. The heart is the most common organ affected by chagas disease. Years to decades after the initial infection, with chronic persistent long-term infection the heart muscle cells are damaged and die. As result of damage, the heart will weaken, enlarge and fail. The heart conduction system that regulates the heartbeat is also damaged leading to an irregular heartbeat. Due to the irregular heartbeat, they may develop dizziness, pass out, and have seizures. Blood clots may occur and lead to stroke. Other organs that are preferentially infected are the food tube, esophagus and large intestine, colon. The esophagus will become weakened and enlarge. As a result, swallowing becomes progressively more difficult, painful with chest pain, coughing, choking on food with vomiting, reflux and pneumonia. There will be weight loss and wasting. The colon likewise will become weakened and enlarged, making defecation more difficult and leading to constipation and abdominal pain. The fatality rate for chagas disease is estimated to be 1%.

Congenital chagas disease will occur when a Trypanosome infected pregnant woman passes the infective parasite form transplacental, resulting in infection to the fetus. She may already be infected with an acute or chronic infection, when she becomes pregnant or alternatively become infected after pregnancy was established. Estimates are that there are at least 2 million females of childbearing potential in Latin America already infected with *Trypanosoma cruzi*. 5 to 12% of infants born to *Trypanosoma cruzi* infected women will develop congenital chagas disease. A pregnant woman with chronic chagas disease may show no symptoms of illness. However, for pregnancy, there is an increased risk of stillbirth, increased chance of a preterm birth or baby with a low birth weight.

As many as 30% of those with congenital chagas disease will at birth have heart muscle inflammation, myocarditis, with progression to life threatening cardiac and digestive disease. They may also have breathing difficulties, brain inflammation, meningoencephalitis, anemia and an enlarged liver and spleen. It is also possible they will show no signs or symptoms of chagas disease until later in childhood. As young adults they may have digestive, neurologic and chronic heart muscle damage with varying degrees of cardiac disease. Infants diagnosed and treated in their first year of life have the best outcome with a nearly 100% cure rate.

The first step in the diagnosis of chagas disease is to consider the potential exposure to *Trypanosoma cruzi* from travel or work in an endemic area. Consider areas where the kissing bug is known to live, the potential for congenital chagas disease or food borne illness. The gold standard for diagnosis of chagas disease whether acute, chronic or congenital has been the identification of the parasite in stained blood smears. Alternatively for those immunosuppressed or immunocompromised, look for parasites in microscopic examination of lymph node or bone marrow aspirates, spinal fluid or fluid from around the heart. Culture or PCR analysis are additional testing measures.

Trypanosoma cruzi may be recovered in a blood culture over the first 60 days after infection. There are several serological tests that measure antibody titers that have been approved for diagnosis of chagas disease. Combining different test measures will increase the accuracy of diagnosing chagas disease. Antibodies from serologic tests may remain positive for a long period of time. For congenital chagas disease, seeing parasites in a blood smear or a positive PCR would be diagnostic. Mother's antibodies may remain detectable in the baby's system for up to 8 to 9 months after birth. If all of these are negative at birth, the child has not acquired chagas disease.

The goal is through treatment to eliminate the parasite and reduce the progression to more serious disease. The earlier the treatment is started the more effective the results. Early treatment may prevent cardiac disease. Treatment in the chronic stage may not completely eradicate the parasite nor stop disease progression, all those with acute chagas disease including congenital chagas disease should be treated as early as possible. Because of the potential of long-term adverse effects, treat all chronically infected individuals up to 18 years of age as well. Any woman of childbearing potential with chagas disease should be treated before she becomes pregnant. Once cardiac changes have begun, treatment of those with chronic chagas disease does not reduce the occurrence of cardiac complications.

There are approved medications that have been shown to be effective in treating chagas disease. The earlier in the course of the illness treatment is initiated, the more effective the results. A limiting factor is that early in the course of the illness there may be few or no symptoms. Benznidazole is the drug of choice for both acute and chronic chagas disease. It has been shown to effectively reduce the duration and severity of the illness. When initiated as early as possible, reports are there will be a 85% overall cure rate for symptoms and 70% parasitological cure. For those 2 years of age and older, it is dosed 2 to 5 up to 7.5 mg/kg/day divided into 2 equal doses given for 30 to 60 days. It may not be used to treat a pregnant woman because it will pass into the placenta and damage the fetus. Side effects of this medication would be nerve inflammation, rash and decreased white blood cell count.

A second medication Nifurtimox also when initiated early will produce an overall 90% cure rate for symptoms and a 70% parasitological cure. Unfortunately, it has a greater number of adverse effects including gastrointestinal upset with vomiting, nausea, pain, loss of appetite and weight, restlessness, seizures, nerve pain and insomnia. Because of its harmful effects, it likewise cannot be given during pregnancy. Adults would receive 8 to 10 mg/kg/day, adolescents would receive 12.5 to 15 mg/kg/day, 1 to 10 years of age would receive 15 to 20 mg/kg/day. For all age groups, dosing will be divided into four equal doses given a day for 90 up to 120 days. Treatment of those with chronic chagas disease has a less than 10% parasitological cure rate. Even with treatment serologic tests, measuring antibodies and PCR measuring parasite DNA may remain positive for a long period of time in part due to a 100% parasitological cure not being achieved. A negative PCR after treatment may suggest a more successful result and parasitological cure.

Individuals with chronic chagas disease should have an electrocardio-gram performed every six months evaluating control of the heart rhythm. If an arrhythmia has developed, these people will benefit from a pacemaker. If the heart shows signs of weakening, enlargement and failure, they should receive appropriate treatment like any other heart patient. Those with progressive esophageal disease may benefit from surgery splitting the esopha-geal muscles to allow easier swallowing. For those with colonic dysfunction, initially they may benefit from dietary changes with increases in fiber, use of laxative and enemas. As the disease progresses with enlargement and dilata-tion of the colon, surgical removal of the area may be of benefit. It is import-ant for people living in endemic areas to be routinely screened and followed for onset of infection or progression of cardiac and gastrointestinal. disease. Begin treatment early, as soon as these changes are noted. Treat women with chagas disease to decrease the chances of congenital infection. Make sure they are not pregnant or become pregnant during the time they are being treated with medication.

Sleeping sickness: African Trypanosomiasis

Sleeping sickness is caused by the protozoan parasite *Trypanosoma brucei*. It occurs only in areas that are infested with the tsetse fly and disease occurs because of a bite by an infected tsetse fly. It has been reported in 36 Sub-Saharan African countries. It may be observed in non-endemic areas like North America, Europe and Australia as a result of visitors to safa-ris, military personnel, immigrants traveling from endemic areas and becom-ing ill in nonendemic areas. There are two unique subtypes of this parasite producing sleeping sickness, *Trypanosoma brucei gambiense* and *Trypanosoma brucei rhodesiense*. *Trypanosoma brucei gambiense* occurs in West and Central Africa. It is responsible for a chronic form of African trypanosomiasis and causes 97% of all cases of sleeping sickness. It now was found mainly in the Democratic Republic of Congo. *Trypanosoma brucei rhodesiense* occurs in East Africa and produces a form of acute African trypanosomiasis. It is responsible for 3% of all cases of sleeping sickness. It is found mainly in Zambia and Malawi. Uganda continues to have both types of trypanosomes.

Trypanosoma brucei has a complex lifecycle and must pass through both a vector and a mammalian host. The tsetse fly becomes infected when feeding on an infected mammal. The trypomastigote stage is taken into the fly during blood feeding. It will develop in the salivary gland of the fly. The infective stage, the trypomastigote, is inoculated by the bite of an infected tsetse fly. It multiplies at the site of infection and forms a red puffy bump; a nodule or ulcer called a chancre. 70 to 90% with rhodesiense will have a skin lesion develop in 3 to 14 days after being bitten by an infected tsetse fly. Fever and parasitemia, parasites in the blood stream, occur around the same time. It will spread through the bloodstream and lymphatic system to different tissues and organs starting the hemolymphatic stage. Symptoms are fever and headache. 50% will develop a rash on their torso with swollen painful lymph occur in the back of the neck.

Chancre rarely occur with *Trypanosoma gambiense*. With *Trypanosoma gambiense* swollen lymph nodes occur in the back of the neck. During this stage parasites are found in the bloodstream and can be aspirated from the lymph nodes. Signs and symptoms subside after this acute first stage. For *Trypanosoma gambiense*, heart inflammation and myocarditis may occur over time. *Trypanosoma rhodesiense* produces a more acute illness with cardiac changes occurring more rapidly. For both types, this initial stage is followed by a second stage with the parasite entering the central nervous system, brain, producing the meningoencephalitis stage. This stage occurs within weeks of the infected bite for *Trypanosoma rhodesiense* and months to years for *Trypanosoma gambiense*. As the disease progresses signs of late-stage illness occur including severe headache, nighttime insomnia, daytime sleepiness, and impaired brain function. There will be progressive brain degeneration due to inflammation resulting in coma and death. *Trypanosoma gambiense* is a slower progressive illness and will have weakness, tremors, confusion, difficulty walking and coordination and dementia. If untreated death may occur 1 to 2 years after onset of neurological symptoms. *Trypanosoma rhodesiense* is more acute and if untreated death may occur within six months after neurological disease has begun.

Diagnostic measures are the same as for chagas disease. Microscopic examination of blood would be the gold standard but there may be few parasites in the bloodstream. During the second stage of illness, parasites may be seen in the cerebral spinal fluid. Serologic tests may be of limited predictive value. Molecular testing including the polymerase chain reaction (PCR) and nucleic acid amplification test (NAAT) are more accurate. It is important to identify the specific subtype to begin the most effective treatment.

The earlier treatment is initiated the more effective and optimal results. Ideally treatment would be started before central nervous system disease, the second stage has begun. Unfortunately, diagnosis is most often delayed until the second stage. For *Trypanosoma gambiense* at its first stage, Pentamidine 4 mg/kg/day intramuscular or intravenous once a day for 7 days would be the drug of choice. *Trypanosoma rhodesiense* at stage one of disease, Suramin 20 mg/kg intravenously on days 1, 3, 6, 14 and 21 after a test dose of 100 mg intravenously would be the drug of choice. If disease has progressed to the second stage, medicines that cross the blood brain barrier and get into the brain must be used. At this stage of illness for *Trypanosoma rhodesiense*, Melarsoprol 2.2 mg/kg/day intravenously for 10 days is the only recommended medication. For second stage *Trypanosoma gambiense*, use Eflornithine 100 mg/kg 4 times a day for 14 days given intravenous or a combination of Nifurtimox 15 mg/kg/day divided into 3 equal doses given intravenously for 10 days with Eflornithine 200 mg/kg twice a day intravenously for 7 days. There are two new drugs, Fexinidazole and Acoziborole may prove to be effective alternatives.

Prevention of African sleeping sickness starts with protection from the tsetse fly bites. Avoid areas that may be infested with tsetse flies, forests, ravines, or savannas. Individuals should wear light-colored clothing that fully covers their body including arms and legs. They should be encouraged to use insecticides. Stay indoors using air conditioning, screens or netting for beds. Measures to control and reduce the number of vectors and carriers are difficult to carry out. Screening, identifying and treating those with trypanosomiasis has reduced the parasite pool and in turn less opportunity for infection.

Chinese or Oriental Liver Fluke

Clonorchiasis
Clonorchis sinensis
Opisthorchis viverrini
Opisthorchis felineus

Clonorchis sinensis is the human liver fluke. It may also infect buffalo, weasels and foxes. *Opisthorchis viverrini* and *Opisthorchis felineus* are dog and cat liver flukes that may also infect people. Infection is acquired by eating raw or undercooked infected freshwater fish and shrimp. More than 100 species of freshwater fish and several species of freshwater shrimp may become infected. These flukes will infect the bile ducts and produce damage to the liver, gall-bladder and their ducts. It is estimated that worldwide 45 up to 200 million people are infected with these liver flukes. As many as 15 million people in China are infected with *Clonorchis*. The infection rate in certain areas of China may range from 17 up to 85%. The occurrence of infection in South Korea may be 2.9% up to 7.4%, 22 up to 85% in Thailand and as high as 37.5% in certain areas of Vietnam.

Liver flukes have a specific range depending upon their snail and freshwater fish and shrimp hosts. *Clonorchis sinensis* occurs in Eastern Europe, Eastern Russia, Manchuria, East Asia, China, Korea, Japan, Vietnam and Taiwan. *Opisthorchis viverrini* occurs in Southeast Asia, Thailand, Lao People's Democratic Republic, Cambodia, Mekong basin and Vietnam with its main reservoir being dogs. Adult liver flukes may produce several thousand eggs per day with *Opisthorchis* as many as 6000 eggs produced and released daily. *Opisthorchis felineus* occurs in Eastern Europe, Southeast Asia, Ukraine, Russia, Byelorussia, Siberia, Italy, Greece and Germany with its main reservoir being cats. Infection occurs in North America from imported infected fresh-water fish and shrimp as well as travelers and immigrants from endemic areas.

For all types of Oriental liver flukes, dogs, cats and pigs may serve as a reservoir, being infected and through defecating return eggs into the environment. These animals may become infected by being fed scraps of infected fish.

Liver fluke eggs are found in the water and are ingested by freshwater snails and certain shrimp. In these hosts the miracidium will hatch out of the egg. The miracidia will penetrate the intestinal wall of the snail or shrimp and form the sporocyst. Sporocysts contain a developmental stage called rediae. Rediae will develop into cercariae. Infection with one egg may end up producing 3700 to 10,000 cercariae that are released into the water. Once cercariae emerge from the snail over the next 72 hours they swim to find a freshwater fish or shrimp. The cercariae will penetrate the skin of the fish or shrimp and in 15 to 20 minutes form a cyst in muscle, the metacercaria stage. Over the next 23 to 30 days the metacercaria continued to develop and become infective. They may remain infective in the fish or shrimp for 30 days up to 1 1/2 years. When raw or undercooked infected fish or shrimp are ingested, trypsin in the small intestine triggers the release of metacercaria. In 9 to 12 minutes these juvenile flukes migrate from the duodenum of the small intestine to the intrahepatic, common bile and pancreatic ducts. Approximately four weeks after infection started, they have developed into egg producing adults. Eggs will pass back into the intestines and are dumped in feces.

Adult *Clonorchis* flukes may be 25 mm long and Opisthorchis adults 12 mm long. They may live 20 up to 30 years. They excrete and secrete products that cause inflammation to the lining of the liver, gallbladder and their ducts and trigger the immune system to produce factors that cause additional damage. As adult worms accumulate, they may also clog the bile ducts causing bile to accumulate in the gallbladder and ducts. As a result, gall stones may develop, and fibrosis and scarring will occur to the liver, gallbladder and bile ducts. The liver and gallbladder will enlarge. Chronic epithelial bile duct inflammation and damage will in time lead to the development of a highly malignant cancer of the bile ducts called cholangiocarcinoma. Estimates are 10% of all *Opisthorchis viverrini* infections will develop cholangiocarcinoma.

Most infections with liver flukes are asymptomatic and discovered incidentally on a routine stool examination. Symptoms may be delayed for decades. Symptoms worsen with both the length of infection and number of adult worms present. Moderate or severe infection may have symptoms develop 2 to 4 weeks after ingestion of the metacercaria. The symptoms would be indigestion, right upper abdominal pain, fever, loss of appetite, headache, nausea, vomiting and diarrhea. Hepatitis will develop from prolonged infection, causing a yellowish color to the skin and eyes. Examination would also show an enlarged liver and spleen.

Diagnosis is confirmed by identifying the proglottids or eggs in the stool. Serology tests could be performed measuring IgG and IgM antibodies. The IgG antibody would confirm that at some point a liver fluke infection occurred. A positive IgM antibody would indicate an ongoing or recent infection. A PCR test on either blood or stool measuring fluke DNA is specific and more accurate for diagnosing infection. Liver enzymes are typically normal, however elevated jaundice markers like bilirubin would be present. One enzyme, alkaline phosphatase may be elevated as well as peripheral blood samples having an elevated number of eosinophil white blood cells. Ultrasound, CT or MRI scan may be performed showing dilated liver, gallbladder and bile ducts with accumulation of bile and gallstones. Signs of cholangiocarcinoma changes may be seen and are consistent with liver fluke infection. Ultrasound may show worms moving around in the gallbladder ducts.

Treatment is with Praziquantel taken orally, 25 mg/kg per dose with three doses a day for two consecutive days. This has been noted to have a 94 to 100% cure rate. Alternatively, Albendazole taken orally, 10 mg/kg/day divided into 2 equal doses for seven days could be used. Maximum Albendazole dose for those weighing 60 kilograms or more is 400 mg twice a day. It has been noted for children that pathological changes in liver, gallbladder and ducts are usually reversed with treatment. Surgery may be done to remove an intraductal carcinoma before it becomes a cholangiocarcinoma.

Prevention would first start with education about how liver flukes are acquired. In many parts of the world eating raw fish and shrimp, sushi, congee, sashimi and koi is both a custom, tradition and perception that it offers health benefits that may be lost by cooking these foods. Metacercaria may unfortunately remain infective on surfaces and objects. Effective handwashing and cleansing of metacercaria contaminated surfaces or objects, knives, cutting boards, dishtowels, contaminated utensils is essential to minimizing exposure and prevent infection. Proper preparation of freshwater fish and shrimp would first start with effective cooking at 63°C, 145°F. This temperature inactivates metacercaria preventing infection. Alternatively freezing at –20°C, –4°F for seven days or –28°C, –18.4°F for 24 hours also prevents infection. Travelers should not eat raw or undercooked freshwater fish or shrimp. Similarly raw or undercooked imported freshwater shrimp or fish should not be eaten.

Cryptosporidium

Cryptosporidiosis
Cryptosporidium parvum
Cryptosporidium hominis

Cryptosporidium is a single cell, intracellular protozoan parasite. It is one of the most common parasitic causes of infectious diarrhea. It has a worldwide distribution but does not occur in Antarctica. Estimates are that in underdeveloped areas of the world as many as 65 up to 97% have *Cryptosporidium* antibodies indicating current or previous infection. Similarly estimates are that 25 up to 65% of people in the United States likewise have positive antibody levels for *Cryptosporidium*. People may acquire infection when traveling to an endemic area but not become symptomatic until returning home.

There are more than 30 different types of *Cryptosporidium* and it occurs in all types of animals, mammals, birds, reptiles and fish. There are 2 specific types that will produce illness in humans, *Cryptosporidium parvum*, and *Cryptosporidium hominis*. *Cryptosporidium hominis* infects people in urban areas and *Cryptosporidium parvum* infects both animals and people in rural areas. Cryptosporidiosis is more likely to cause illness during rainy seasons.

Infection begins when the infective oocysts are orally ingested from fecally contaminated hands, water or food. It may only require as few as 32 oocysts of *Cryptosporidium parvum* and only 10 to 83 oocysts of *Cryptosporidium hominis* to cause infection. During infection it may produce and release as many as 1 billion oocysts from an infected host. The oocysts pass into the small and large intestines where each release 4 sporozoites. The sporozoites attach and burrow into the epithelial lining cells producing inflammation, injury and malabsorption. The sporozoites mature into merozoites that are released back into the intestines. The merozoites differentiate into male and female gametes that fuse and form new oocysts. Thin-walled oocysts may penetrate the intestinal lining producing continued, autoinfection or reinfection. Thick-walled oocysts may pass through the stool into the environment. They are very hardy and resistant, allowing them to survive for months in changing environmental conditions.

Water is the prime source for acquiring the parasite. Water sources that may be contaminated are drinking water, recreational activity water like fountains, swimming pools, water parks and water play areas. Other water sources that may be contaminated are lakes, creeks, ponds or rivers. As much as 65 to 97% of all surface water may be contaminated with *Cryptosporidium*. Surface water may become contaminated from infected animal or human fecal waste passing into the water. Contamination by animal feces, especially from cattle, occurs in farming areas where municipal water depends upon surface water as its source. For this reason, water borne outbreaks of *Cryptosporidium* illness may affect large populations and have occurred in areas of Oregon and Milwaukee.

People living together in overcrowded situations, children in day care and their adult caretakers promote person-to-person spread. Overall poor sanitation conditions create the opportunity for spread of infection. Exposure to contamination from infected animals is another source of infection putting anyone working with animals like veterinarians and vet techs at high risk for *Cryptosporidium* infection.

The incubation period, time from acquisition of oocysts until onset of symptoms is around 8 days. Infection results in inflammation and disruption of the function of the intestinal tract involving both small and large intestines. This results in gastrointestinal symptoms of diarrhea and cramping. It may additionally spread to the gallbladder, pancreas and respiratory tract. Oocysts have been found in sputum and nasal respiratory secretions. They may be aerosolized during coughing. It is unclear if they actively colonize the respiratory tract and its overall significance in transmission of infection. The recovery of oocysts in secretions may only be coincidental and not indicate an active ongoing site of infection.

Cryptosporidium diarrhea unfortunately may last for months to years. Other symptoms may be fever, headache, joint pain (knees, ankles, feet), weight loss, fatigue, nausea and eye pain. The joint pain may begin or last several months after infection started and is the result of the immune system being activated. Abdominal pain and diarrhea may become chronic. *Cryptosporidium* most likely occurs in children under five years of age especially in those less than two years of age. Healthy individuals have varying degrees of diarrhea which may be mild, moderate or severe. Chronic or severe diarrhea may lead to malnutrition.

Children with disorders impairing their immune system function, either immunocompromised or immunosuppressed due to a congenital, genetic or acquired cause will have more severe disease. Those with infections like HIV or organ transplantation may have symptoms that become chronic, more severe and even life-threatening. It is the severe fluid and electrolyte loss through diarrhea that may become life-threatening especially for any child who is immunosuppressed or immunocompromised. Estimates are that worldwide there are annually 202,000 deaths from *Cryptosporidium* infections.

Food may become contaminated through its preparation by infected food handlers especially in a cafeteria setting. Foods that may become naturally contaminated would-be apple cider, raw or unpasteurized goat or cow milk and any foods grown at ground level like strawberries that may be contaminated by animal feces in surface water. Infected workers collecting the produce are another source of contamination.

The gold standard for diagnosis of *Cryptosporidium* is observing oocysts in the stool. The modified Ziehl Nielsen stain or Acid-Fast stain helps to visualize parasites in the stool. Visualizing parasites in the stool is very imprecise and other testing measures are more accurate. Additional diagnostic tests would be serology tests measuring antibodies in the blood and molecular tests like the polymerase chain reaction (PCR) or nuclear amplification test (NAAT) measuring parasite DNA in the stool. Serology tests may show infection in the past with a positive IgG antibody titer and an ongoing or recent infection with a positive IgM antibody titer. The molecular tests have the added benefit of differentiating between *Cryptosporidium parvum* and *Cryptosporidium hominis*. Identification of the specific species may help to determine the source and location of where the infection was acquired.

The mainstay of treatment is supportive care. Most of those with cryptosporidiosis have mild to moderate symptoms and are able to drink enough oral electrolyte solutions to keep up with their gastrointestinal fluid losses. The use of probiotics helps to reestablish the healthy gut status and zinc supplements have been shown to promote healing of the inflamed intestinal tract. Children with a healthy immune system may have spontaneous recovery from *Cryptosporidium*. They may have no more symptoms (clinical cure) in days to weeks and no more oocysts shedding (parasitological cure) in weeks to months. Further additional infections tend to be milder and more self-limited. Reinfection may still occur from oocysts already in the gastrointestinal tract or from the new intake or ingestion of oocysts.

If individuals have symptoms that are severe or persistent for weeks, they may need treatment especially if they have an impaired immune system function. To improve their response to treatment, it may be necessary to try to correct the underlying immune deficiency. If a person has underlying HIV, treat it with ART, otherwise they generally have a poor outcome. If fluid loss is severe, intravenous electrolyte solution may be needed for both fluid and electrolyte replacement. Loperamide may be used for diarrhea control. If symptoms are severe or persistent, they may interfere with the quality of life and school or day care attendance. There are specific recommendations for the use of medications for cryptosporidiosis.

For healthy children with cryptosporidiosis, if diarrhea lasts for more than 2 weeks Nitazoxanide is given orally for 3 days. For those 1 to 3 years of age, they receive 100 mg twice a day. Those 4 to 11 years of age receive 200 mg twice a day. Those 12 years of age and older receive 500 mg twice a day. With treatment, in 3 to 4 days diarrhea resolves and 75% have no oocysts shedding. If Nitazoxanide is not available or not tolerated, the next best option is Paromomycin dosed at 25 to 35 mg/kg/da. It is not specifically approved for treatment of *Cryptosporidium*.

For those with an impaired immune system function, the recommended dosing for these medications is not very effective. Preferably a 2-to-8-week course of Nitazoxanide is used for those with HIV. Children with immunosuppression or immunocompromise 1 to 3 years of age would receive Nitazoxanide 200 mg twice a day. Those 4 to 11 years of age would receive 400 mg twice a day. The combination of Rifaximin and Rifabutin may produce some benefits. Paromomycin has no effect on oocyst shedding in the stool or diarrhea. A combination of Nitazoxanide, Paromomycin and Azithromycin given daily for a month has been used to treat these children. If the child has had an organ transplant and is on antirejection medicine, use Nitazoxanide for at least 2 weeks. Dosing for children 1 to 3 years of age is 100 mg twice a day, 4 to 11 years 200 mg twice a day, those 12 years of age and older would receive 500 up to 1000 mg twice a day.

If diarrhea persists after treatment with Nitazoxanide, recheck the stool for oocysts by microscopic examination and PCR. If oocysts are still present, then treat them with a combination of Nitazoxanide and Paromomycin. Other symptoms, joint pain, eye pain and headache may persist up to two years after the infection has been treated. These symptoms are most likely the result of the immune system activation producing inflammation and damage to these areas and not related to either side effects or the effectiveness of these medications in treating *Cryptosporidium*.

It is unknown how long protection lasts after infection. There is no effective vaccination for *Cryptosporidium*. Control measures consist of effective handwashing with soap. Hand sanitizers are ineffective. The mechanical action of scrubbing the hands helps to physically remove the oocysts from the skin. The oocyst has a thick cellular wall and is resistant to chemical agents. They are not killed by chlorine, bleach or iodine. Hydrogen peroxide may work best for disinfecting and cleaning the hands and surfaces. There should be proper disposal of contaminated material. Wash all foods and produce thoroughly with safe, clean water before consumption. Oocysts may be killed by freezing and cooking or boiling water before its consumption. Maintain safe drinking water through surveillance and monitoring. A small filter pore size less than 5 microns is required for trapping the parasite during the purification of municipal and bottled water. It may be killed by high UV doses, low-power UV light cannot penetrate the oocyst wall and is ineffective.

Dientamoeba fragilis

Dientamoeba fragilis has long been considered to be a nonpathogenic parasite that harmlessly colonizes the gastrointestinal tract. It has been overall forgotten and neglected for its properties and potential to produce illness in people. Because it has not been considered to be pathogenic, it has been poorly studied and investigated with only incomplete information known about its life cycle. In addition to people, wild monkeys in the Philippines, macaques, baboons, gorillas, pigs, and rodents are additional natural hosts.

Dientamoeba fragilis is a flagellate protozoan. It has a worldwide distribution and has been found anywhere that is inhabited by people. The worldwide occurrence ranges from 0.4 to 71% and is believed to have the highest rate found in crowded living conditions and those in close contacts in families. Other reports are that it is more likely to occur in high income areas. This may mean it is prevalent essentially in all groups in all conditions.

Dientamoeba has a high rate of occurrence in healthy populations with no symptoms. Its rate of recovery is reported to be 14.8% in the Netherlands, 6.3% in Belgium, 11.7% in Sweden, 16.9% in the British Isles, 8.8% in Turkey, 4.1% in Italy, 1.5 to 16.8% in Australia, 15.2% in Israel, 8.5% of hospitalized children in Portugal, 0.4 to 24% of children and 2 to 9% of adults in Spain and 1.6 to 83% in Europe. Specifically for those healthy, 25.7 to 37.3% of all ages in Europe and 87 to 100% of children in Canada have *Dientamoeba*. In the United States the prevalence is estimated to be between 1.3 and 21%. It may be contracted through oral ingestion of fecally contaminated food, water or contaminated hands from poor hygiene.

For years only the trophozoite stage was known, but more recently a cyst and precyst form have been identified. They may have an important and specific role in its lifecycle and contagiousness. There is information that

Dientamoeba may be transmitted along with pinworm eggs with *Dientamoeba fragilis* DNA recovered from the core of the pinworm egg.

The role for all three stages, trophozoites, pre-cysts and cysts regarding resistance to environmental changes and contagiousness is unclear. Cysts and pre-cysts may be resistant forms that survive varying environmental conditions. Once trophozoites, cysts or pre-cysts are orally ingested they pass into the large intestines, replicate and produce inflammation in the bowel wall. This may lead to the development of symptoms.

Symptoms may include intermittent diarrhea, nausea, vomiting, abdominal pain, gas, malaise, loss of appetite, poor weight gain and fatigue. Up to 32% may have chronic diarrhea. *Dientamoeba* may be connected to chronic abdominal pain and irritable bowel syndrome. People who have *Dientamoeba* and these symptoms have resolution of symptoms when *Dientamoeba* is treated. For those symptomatic and not treated, symptoms may persist for several years. Alternatively, it is possible that infected individuals may be asymptomatic, symptom free carriers and not have chronic abdominal pain or irritable bowel syndrome symptoms.

Diagnosis is through stool evaluation showing *Dientamoeba* forms microscopically and *Dientamoeba fragilis* DNA through a PCR test. A stool culture for *Dientamoeba* may grow trophozoites. Trophozoites may be shed intermittently so multiple stool samples may be required for analysis. Serology blood test measuring specific IgG and IgM antibodies may be positive for *Dientamoeba*. More than 50% of those with *Dientamoeba* will have a high eosinophil count in their peripheral blood.

Estimates are that without treatment there is a high rate of spontaneous cure, 49 to 100% for children and 57 to 90% for adults. For individuals who continue to have symptoms and *Dientamoeba* has been identified in their stool, treatment is indicated. Both Metronidazole and Paromomycin have been successfully used to treat Dientamoeba.

Paromomycin is given 500 mg orally three times a day for seven days or for the younger age population 25 to 35 mg/kg/da orally divided into 3 doses a day for 4 to 5 up to 7 days. This may produce a 100% cure. Alternatively, Metronidazole 400 to 750 mg three times a day for 3 to 10 days or 20 to 40 mg/kg/day divided into 3 doses a day for 10 days produces an 82 to 100% cure rate. Other information reports that Paromomycin has an 81.8% cure rate compared to 65.4% cure rate for Metronidazole. Considering efficacy and tolerability, Paromomycin appears to be a superior product.

However, if a relapse occurs after a course of Paromomycin, give a 10-day course of Metronidazole.

There is no vaccination for *Dientamoeba fragilis*. The keys to prevention are good hygiene measures, using clean drinking water and prevent fecal contamination of foods and water. Raw vegetables and fruits should be washed with safe, clean water before being eaten.

Dog Heartworm. Dirofilariasis

Dirofilaria immitis
Dirofilaria repens

Dirofilaria immitis and *Dirofilaria repens* are better known as the dog heart-worm. They are nematodes, round worms. They produce infection in their natural hosts, dogs, cats, black bears, foxes, ferrets, otters, ocelots, sea lions and wolves. Dogs and cats cannot directly transmit *Dirofilaria* to humans. Humans are accidentally infected through the bite of an infected mosquito. This is a dead end for this parasite, it cannot undergo its normal development and complete its lifecycle in humans. *Dirofilaria* is more likely to occur in the Western Hemisphere and Asia. It does not routinely occur in Europe or Africa. There are reports of it occurring in Mediterranean areas of France, Italy, Greece and Spain.

Infections are more likely to occur in the Southern and Southeastern United States especially along the Gulf and Atlantic Coasts and the Mississippi River basin. Testing shows that as many as 40% of all dogs more than six months of age in South Texas are positive for *Dirofilaria*. In the United States, 1.1 to 14% of all cats are likewise positive for *Dirofilaria*. In Canada, less than 1% of dogs and 0.4% of cats are infected. The prevalence in people probably mirrors the occurrence in dogs. However, most cases in people are asymptomatic remain undiagnosed resulting in the true incidence being underestimated.

Infected mosquitoes through feeding will introduce the infectious L3 microfilaria stage into animals or people. In animals the larvae will migrate through tissues into the bloodstream. During this migration they mature into adult worms. They pass into the heart and out into the pulmonary artery and pulmonary (lung) blood vessels. From there adult worms will produce and release the L1 larvae into the bloodstream which may be ingested by mosquitoes during a blood meal. In the mosquito the L1 larvae over 14 days will pass through 2 developmental stages, molts, and form the L3 infectious larvae. This stage will pass back into the feeding apparatus of the mosquito and during its next meal will pass to a new host.

If the next host is a human, most of the L3 microfilariae will die during their passage through the subcutaneous tissues. Some may reach the blood system and migrate to the heart. During this transit they also will develop into adults. The adults will pass from the heart into the pulmonary artery and vessels. However, in the human host the adult worms are sterile and produce no L1 larvae. In time adults will die, triggering a response from the immune system. The immune system will produce a wall around the dead or dying worm, forming a granuloma. Dying larvae in the subcutaneous tissue result in formation of abscesses or granulomas.

As many as 50 to 62% of people infected with *Dirofilaria* have no symptoms. In most cases spread of the parasite is limited to the heart and lungs. In the lungs, the adult may lodge in the pulmonary artery. This may lead to inflammation and blockage resulting in the immune system producing a nodule or granuloma. When symptomatic, the most common complaints are chest pain, lung inflammation causing cough, coughing up blood, low-grade fever, chills and malaise. With heart involvement, there may be enlargement of the right ventricle and possible heart failure. Children with a positive test for *Dirofilaria* are more likely to also have allergies, rhinitis and asthma. *Dirofilaria* may pass into the eye involving the eyeball or surrounding areas. Depending on its position it may be possible to visualize the worm just under the outer layer of the eyeball. Complete surgical removal of the worm is necessary. If part of the worm remains or the worm should die in this area it will trigger the body's immune response creating eye damage, visual impairment and blindness.

Definitive diagnosis is through surgical removal of a nodule reserved followed by examination showing the worm. Surgical removal of a nodule is reserved for the most severe cases. 5 to 10% will have an increased number of eosinophils in their peripheral blood sample. A PCR test on the removed or needle aspirated nodule may show *Dirofilaria* DNA. PCR on blood or serology tests measuring IgG and IgM antibodies have been unreliable and overall have not proven to be useful. Newer assay measures may be more accurate.

Surgical removal of a nodule is curative. Those who have complications or have a heavy or high number of infectious larvae may need to be treated with antiparasitic medications. They could receive Doxycycline with or without Ivermectin. Diethylcarbamazine has been used as a successful alternative.

These medications are given to reduce cardiovascular effects or to eliminate a symbiotic germ *Wolbachia* that is in *Dirofilaria* and necessary for its survival. Medications may kill the larvae passing through the subcutaneous tissue and lymphatic system but have no effect on the established adult worms. Reducing the number of mosquitoes in areas of high disease, endemic areas, will minimize infections.

Dog Tapeworm

Dipylidium caninum

Dipylidium caninum is the dog tapeworm but is a common cause of infection in people, especially in children who have close contact with domesticated and free range dogs and cats. It has a worldwide distribution occurring in Europe, Asia and the Americas. Specifically, it has been reported in Italy, Poland, Germany, Bulgaria, Romania, Turkey, Spain, England, the United States, Canada, Japan, the Philippines, China, India, Sri Lanka, Brazil, Mexico, Chile, Uruguay, Argentina, Guatemala, Puerto Rico, South Africa and Australia. Infants and young children most likely acquire the dog tapeworm due to playing with or in close contact with dogs and their own poor personal hygiene. Animals will groom themselves and have fleas around their mouth and face. The fleas may be infected with *Dipylidium caninum* larvae. Additionally cat fleas, human fleas or the chewing louse of dogs may similarly be infected by dog tapeworm larvae. Kids may incidentally ingest infected fleas by kissing on or by being licked by dogs and cats.

The infection rate in dogs and cats ranges between 1 to 60%. Estimates are that in the United States 50% of all dogs are infected with dog tapeworm. In Mexico the infection rate for dogs is between 34 and 54%. In Spain, 3% of all dogs and 33% of all cats are infected with *Dipylidium caninum*. The adult stage of the dog tapeworm will be in the host small intestines. Segments of the tapeworm called proglottids contain eggs and will break off from the end of the tapeworm and either crawl or be passed in the feces. In the soil the proglottids rupture releasing the eggs. The eggs are ingested by fleas. In the flea intestine the egg releases the oncosphere stage. Alternatively, eggs may be on an animal's fur from proglottids rupturing in the gastrointestinal tract. Fleas may directly feed on these eggs setting the sequence in motion for continued larvae development. The oncosphere will then pass into the flea's body cavity and develop into the cysticercoid larval stage. About 36 hours after the flea takes a blood meal, the cysticercoid develops into the infective metacestode stage.

When dogs, cats or children accidentally ingest the flea containing the metacestode larval stage, it will pass into the intestines and develop into the adult tapeworm. It may take 3 to 4 weeks after the beginning of infection with ingestion of infected fleas until mature adults have developed. The adult may reach 15 to 60 cm (6 to nearly 24 inches) in length. Infected children may have anywhere from one up to as many as 50 *Dipylidium caninum* adult worms in their intestines. The parasite load is the result of the number of infected fleas ingested and number of infective metacestode larvae in each ingested flea.

Most infections are asymptomatic. When symptoms occur, the child may have mild abdominal pain, bloating, loss of appetite, irritability, agitation, restlessness, poor sleep, anal itching and pain, hives, vomiting, constipation and diarrhea.

Diagnosis of dog tapeworm is made by visualizing the proglottids with or without their structurally identified eggs in a fecal sample. It would be unusual to visualize eggs in the feces unless the proglottids had ruptured. Eggs in this free state are rarely seen in infected feces. They are not very stable and quickly disintegrate. The proglottids are the size and shape of a poppyseed when dry and look more like a cucumber seed when wet. In the stool they may also look like grains of rice or sesame seeds. Examination of a peripheral blood smear would show an increased number of eosinophils. A PCR test on feces would show dog tapeworm DNA.

Dog tapeworm infections in children usually resolve spontaneously in six weeks without complications. However symptomatic infection may persist up to one year. If a child is having prolonged or exaggerated unacceptable symptoms, the medicine of choice to treat dog tapeworm infection is a single dose of Praziquantel 5 to 20 mg/kg given orally. In heavy infections a second dose 2 to 4 weeks after the first dose may be necessary. Praziquantel would also be used to treat dog tapeworm infection in dogs and cats. Other alternatives would be Albendazole and Thiabendazole, but they are not as effective.

Optimal prevention would involve flea and lice control. On a regular basis check pet fecal samples for worm infestation and treat them when they are present. Combine flea control with treatment of adult worms to break the lifecycle for dog tapeworm. Proper disposal of dog and cat feces is also important in breaking the lifecycle by removing proglottids and eggs from the soil. Flea control measures with protecting animals year around with an oral or topical product in addition to environmental control for flea exposure are essential.

Dwarf Tapeworm. Rat Tapeworm

Hymenolepis
Hymenolepiasis
Hymenolepis nana **(Dwarf tapeworm),**
   Hymenolepis diminuta **(Rat tapeworm)**

There are 2 species of Hymenolepis that are important for people, *nana* and *diminuta*. They have a wide distribution. They occur in both humans and rodents, mice and rats. *Hymenolepis* is the most common tapeworm (cestode) in the world. It prefers dry, warm areas of the world. Estimates are that 0.5 to 5% in Europe, 0.2 to 28% in Asia, 0.9 to 23% in the Americas and 1.8 to 2.9% in Africa are infected with *Hymenolepis*.

In some areas of the world 17.5 to 25% of all children and worldwide 50 to 75 million people have *Hymenolepis nana* (dwarf tapeworm) infection. It is prevalent in Africa, Latin America and India. Poor personal hygiene and crowding like in daycares and schools are risk factors for its transmission. According to the World Health Organization hotspots for *Hymenolepis nana* are Mexico, Brazil, Peru, Afghanistan, Ethiopia, Egypt, Pakistan, India, Bangladesh, and Lao People's Democratic Republic. More specific breakdown estimates are 33% of those in the Sudan, 10% in Ethiopia, 9% in Argentina, and nearly 8% in India are infected with *Hymenolepis nana*. In the United States, Kentucky had a 1% and North Carolina a 3% incidence in the 1930's.

Human infections with *Hymenolepis diminuta* (rat tapeworm) have been reported in 80 countries around the world including Southeast Asia, the Americas and Eastern Mediterranean. Hotspots are Costa Rica and Brazil. Previous data had shown the United States to be a hotspot with 1930's data reporting Kentucky and North Carolina having a 0.03% incidence and the most recent data showed a 1% occurrence for the United States and 0.1% in Canada. Today cases are overall more likely to occur in Bangladesh, Afghanistan and Brazil.

Hymenolepis nana requires no intermediate host. It may be passed from one person to another by hand to mouth transmission. Food handlers that work with food processing could be a common source for *Hymenolepis nana*. They could be directly or indirectly transmitted through food to places where food is prepared and served. Greeting by shaking hands, especially if not washing hands after defecation and not washing raw vegetables before consumption promotes the spread of *Hymenolepis nana*.

Alternatively, *Hymenolepis nana* may be contracted by ingestion of food or water contaminated with its eggs. The ingested eggs release motile embryos, the oncospheres. They invade the lining of the small intestine and encyst in the intestinal villi. In 3 to 4 days, they develop into the cysticercoid that invaginates destroying the intestinal lining. Within 96 hours the cysticercoid then breaks out of the lining into the inside of the intestines and in about 1 month develops into the adult tapeworm.

Hymenolepis nana eggs are in the last or terminal segment of the adult worm that breaks off into the gastrointestinal tract. This segment is called a gravid proglottid and will disintegrate releasing the infective eggs before being passed in the feces. These infected eggs may penetrate the intestinal lining and undergo the process of developing into adults. From the time an egg is produced until maturation to an adult worm may be 3 to 4 weeks. Infection may build rapidly in a child due to this autoinfection route. However, outside a human host, *Hymenolepis nana* eggs cannot survive in the environment for more than two weeks.

Most infections are asymptomatic. However, it is estimated that infections with more than 10 worms will produce symptoms. Presumptively the heavier the worm burden (lots of worms in the gastrointestinal tract) the worse the symptoms. The symptoms would be abdominal pain, nausea, vomiting, diarrhea, fever, fatigue, loss of appetite, weakness, anemia, impaired growth with poor weight gain, anal itching, irritability, behavioral changes, sleep problems and anemia causing headache and dizziness. Death has been reported when *Hymenolepis nana* infections occur in immunocompromised patients. In an immunocompromised individual there may be abnormal even malignant parasite development, disseminated disease and death.

Hymenolepis nana is the only cestode that may be spread person-to-person as well as autoinfection. Rats and mice in the wild or pets (like gerbils) may transmit *Hymenolepis nana* by ingesting infected human feces or *Hymenolepis diminuta* by ingesting infected specific types of insects called arthropods. *Hymenolepis diminuta* (the rat tapeworm) does require an intermediate insect host for making the cysticercoid stage. In some areas up to 60% of all rodents are infected with *Hymenolepis nana* and 0.5 up to 33% may be infected with *Hymenolepis diminuta*. The cysticercoid stage is found in the small intestine of rodents. Its eggs, when ingested by feces eating arthropods develop into the cysticercoid larva. Rodents then ingest the infected arthropod.

Children may be accidentally infected by ingesting an infected arthropod. When the infected arthropod is eaten by a rodent or child, the cysticercoid larvae will develop into an adult worm in their intestines. Its eggs may be ingested in food or water contaminated with infected insects or mice and rat feces. Insects such as fleas, grain beetles, flour weevils, cockroaches and flour moths may be accidentally ingested in different foods like flour, meal, and cereal products. These may contain infected insects or rodent feces contaminated with *Hymenolepis* eggs*. As described the eggs develop into the cysticercoid stage. The cysticercoid stage is then released by digestion of the infected arthropod. It attaches to the wall of the small intestine and in 2 to 3 weeks matures into an adult worm. *Hymenolepis nana* adults are 15 to 40 millimeters long (up to 1.5 inches) and *Hymenolepis diminuta* 20 to 60 centimeters long (7 1/2 up to 23 inches). Adults may live for years in the intestinal tract of both humans and rodents.

Diagnosis is made by identifying its eggs in the stool. The eggs of *Hymenolepis nana* and *diminuta* each have unique characteristic features allowing their specific identification and differentiation. A serology blood test may be completed to identify antibodies against *Hymenolepis*. This test is nonspecific and not able to differentiate between *Hymenolepis nana* and *Hymenolepis diminuta*. DNA PCR test on feces is more specific and may be done to identify *Hymenolepis nana* or *Hymenolepis diminuta*. A complete blood count could show an increase in a cell type called eosinophils which may be seen with parasitic infections. There may be signs of anemia with folate and B12 deficiency.

Different medications are used to kill *Hymenolepis* tapeworms. Niclosamide kills the worms and is given 40 mg/kg for a one-time dose. Other Niclosamide doses used would be 1 gram first day single dose then a 500 mg single dose for the next six days, or 2 gm first day dose then 1 gm once a day for an additional five days. Praziquantel kills the tapeworm by paralyzing it and is given as a 25 mg/kg one time dose. Alternative treatments with Praziquantel would be a single 10 mg/kg daily dose for seven days or 20 mg/kg single daily dose for five days. Treatment combining Praziquantel and Nicolsamide has an efficacy of more than 90%. Nitazoxanide given as a single 500 mg daily dose for three days has been shown to be 75 to 93% effective. Another treatment is Albendazole dosed at 400 mg a day for three days or 800 mg a day for three days then repeat the dosing in seven days. Niclosamide has been used when there is ongoing neurological disease.

* As a side note, our foods can also have fly eggs, rodent feces and insect parts. This is allowable by certain FDA guidelines that recognize that these are natural, unavoidable contaminants in our food that occur during the growing, processing and packaging of food. The FDA considers certain specified levels to be safe and not present a risk for our health. See the FDA's "Food Defect Levels Handbook". This makes you wonder not only in the United States but how much of the population in developed countries are naturally infected by an array of parasites transmitted in our foods and its impact on the occurrence of chronic, non-life-threatening, annoying symptoms like recurrent abdominal pain or recurrent episodes of nausea and/or vomiting.

Echinostoma

Echinostomiasis
Echinostoma more than 120 species

Echinostoma is an intestinal trematode of aquatic birds and mammals. It has a worldwide distribution with now more than 120 different species identified. It is found in Asia and Oceana, Europe and America. Specific countries are Thailand, China, Taiwan, Indonesia, Cambodia, Malaysia, South Korea, India, Nepal, the Philippines, Kenya, Tanzania and North America. Estimates are that more than 50 million people worldwide are infected with *Echinostoma*. Specific breakdown of prevalence in different geographic areas would include 7.5 to 22.4% of those children in Cambodia have *Echinostoma*. Taiwan has an occurrence of 2.8 up to 6.5%, for all ages in Cambodia 2.4 up to 7.5%, Northern Luzon 7 up to 17%, Southern Philippines for those 15 to 30 years of age have a 55% occurrence of *Echinostoma* and parts of Korea have a 22% occurrence. Thailand has a reported prevalence of 55% and over 50% of those in Laos and Vietnam have *Echinostoma* infection. It may be imported to different parts of the world through immigrants, refugees and travelers.

It is spread by fecal contamination of unembryonated eggs in freshwater ponds, lakes, streams and imported infected food. When these eggs contact freshwater, they become embryonated (fertile) and hatch releasing the miracidia. This is the free-swimming form and will seek out specific snails. In the snail the miracidia develop into the sporocyst stage, multiply and finally develop into the cercariae. The cercariae are released into the water. They are free swimming, seek out and penetrate clams, various snails, fish, salamanders, tadpoles and frogs. In these hosts they develop into metacercaria. Alternatively, cercariae may remain in the initial snail host and develop into metacercaria. Metacercaria are the infective stage for mammals and aquatic birds. Once a mammal ingests an infected snail, clam, fish or frog, the metacercariae will excyst in the intestines and develop into adult worms. Adult worms produce and release eggs that pass in the feces into the environment. They are viable and with favorable environmental conditions may survive and hatch over five months.

Most cases are mild and have no symptoms. However, metacercaria and adult worms may cause abdominal pain that may be severe, diarrhea, fatigue and malnutrition. Heavy worm loads may cause intestinal perforation and serious anemia.

Diagnosis is through microscopic examination of feces showing *Echinostoma* eggs. It is possible to collect and identify adult worms in the feces. Serology test may identify the IgG antibody and indicate an infection at some point in time or IgM antibody consistent with an ongoing or recent infection. A PCR test on stool is a more accurate way of identifying ongoing *Echinostoma* infection.

Treatment is with a single dose of Praziquantel 25 to 40 mg/kg as a single dose with a 100% cure rate.

There is no effective vaccination for *Echinostoma*. It's more likely to occur in areas of poor sanitation. The first step in reducing its occurrence is to protect the water from fecal contamination with proper sanitation and the availability of clean drinking water. Additional measures would be to educate people not to ingest raw, uncooked or pickled freshwater aquatic clams, snails, fish, or frogs.

Elephantiasis. Lymphatic Filariasis

Wuchereria bancrofti
Brugia malayi
Brugia timori

Wuchereria bancrofti is a nematode parasite with a complex lifecycle transmitted by the bite of a nighttime feeding mosquito. It will produce irreversible and debilitating disease. It affects more than 150 million people worldwide in 83 developing countries, tropics, subtropics, the West Indies, Northern Africa, India, certain South Pacific Islands, American Samoa, Southeast Asia, areas of Central and South America and Latin America. It does not naturally occur in Europe and North America, but cases may occur there due to visits by travelers, immigrants and refugees from endemic areas of the world resulting in "imported infections". The last natural infection case in the United States was in the early 20th century in Charleston, South Carolina.

Other lymphatic filaria are *Brugia malayi* (Southeast Asia, the Philippines, Korea, Japan) and *Brugia timori* (Southeast Indonesia and islands of the lesser Sunda Archipelago, Timor, Sumba, Lembata, Panta and Alor).

Children will become infected with *Wuchereria* when a mosquito carrying the larval L3 stage takes a blood meal. Multiple infected mosquito bites may be required to develop lymphatic filariasis. Short-term exposure in endemic areas carries little risk. The larvae enter the skin and develop into the adult worm in the lymphatic system causing swelling in the extremities and for males swelling the scrotum. Swelling may also occur in the breasts. The female worm over the next 5 to 8 years produces millions of microfilariae that migrate from the lymphatic system to the surrounding blood vessels. There they are ingested by mosquitoes taking a blood meal.

Microfilariae taken in during a blood meal will pass into the mosquito's midgut, penetrate and pass through its wall, then migrate to the chest muscles. In the chest muscles it will undergo two additional developmental stages producing the infective L3 stage that migrates to the mosquito feeding apparatus, the proboscis. The next round of transmission occurs with infected mosquito feeding.

Infection may occur early in life, but symptoms may be delayed until puberty or early adulthood. Individuals may remain asymptomatic carriers with no or minimal symptoms. However, everyone infected with *Wuchereria* will have kidney and lymphatic system damage. Estimates are that approximately one third of all those infected will become symptomatic with tissue swelling (lymphedema), hydrocele (swelling of the scrotum) and thickening and hardening of the skin. These symptoms combine to make a disorder called "elephantiasis".

As many as 40 million people may have elephantiasis. It is more likely to occur with chronic or reinfection. As a result of secondary bacterial infection, episodes of fever, inflamed tender swollen lymph nodes in the groin and armpit area and swelling to the effected extremities of the body may occur. Adult worms and microfilariae killed by the body's immune system are toxic and will cause inflammation and damage to the body.

Diagnosis is made through clinical examination of the individual and microscopic detection of microfilariae in a Giemsa-stained blood smear collected between 10 PM and 2 AM. Serologic blood test measuring antibody levels may determine infection at some point but unless IgM antibody is positive would not be consistent with ongoing infection. A PCR test on a blood sample is more accurate showing parasite DNA in the bloodstream.

For treatment, an individual could receive Diethylcarbamazine dosed at 1mg/kg as a single oral dose on day 1; the dose on day 2 is 1 mg/kg given orally 3 times a day; 1–2 mg/kg orally 3 times a day on day 3; 2 mg/kg 3 times a day orally on days 4 through 14. When given in combination with Albendazole it is dosed as a 6 mg/kg single-dose or if younger than nine years of age give this dose for a 12-day course. Alternatively, Albendazole may be dosed 15 mg/kg/da as a single daily oral dose with a maximum dose of 400 mg for 3 to 28 days. These may be given along with Doxycycline 100 mg twice a day for four weeks and intravenous Ivermectin. Diethylcarbamazine is geared more for killing microfilariae but will also kill a portion of the adults. Albendazole also kills microfilariae. Doxycycline will target and kill *Wolbachia*, a bacterium in the worms that is essential for their survival.

For those with a high microfilariae and worm load, treatment killing a large number at one time will produce a high amount of different toxic products from dead parasites. This may cause fever, generalized body ache, itching, low blood pressure and when severe death. To minimize these adverse events, when initiating treatment give antihistamine and steroid to block or reduce these adverse toxic reactions from the killed worms and microfilariae. There is no cure or specific drug therapy for lymphedema.

Fibrosis and scarring are considered irreversible and are currently treated with supportive measures. However, there are reports that with combination therapy and early treatment elephantiasis is 100% curable. The overall goal is to keep the area clean and dry to prevent secondary bacterial infection. A hydrocele would be treated with surgery.

Brugia infections are usually asymptomatic. However, it may cause a similar but milder illness compared to *Wuchereria*. It is more likely to involve the upper extremities. It is spread through the bite of a *Brugia* infected mosquito. It goes through the same developmental stages as *Wuchereria*. Adults in the lymphatic system will cause inflammation and obstruction of these channels. Scarring of the lymphatics along with swelling which may be substantial will cause elephantiasis.

Diagnosis of *Brugia* would also be through visualization of its microfilariae in a blood smear stained with Giemsa and measuring antibodies or a positive PCR test. Diethylcarbamazine is the drug of choice for treatment for *Brugia* infection. Doxycycline 100 mg a day may be combined with Diethylcarbamazine and Albendazole or given singly over six weeks to kill *Brugia* microfilariae.

There is no vaccination for the lymphatic filariasis. Prevent mosquito bites by wearing long sleeves and pants when outdoors between dusk and dawn. Apply an effective mosquito repellent to exposed skin areas. Clothes may be washed in a Permethrin detergent which is an effective insect repellent. For indoor nighttime protection, sleep in air-conditioning, screened windows or under a mosquito net treated with Permethrin.

Endolimax

Endolimax nana

Endolimax nana is an ameba protozoan. It has a worldwide distribution with an estimated 950 million healthy individuals having *Endolimax nana*. It typically occurs in areas of poor sanitation. The breakdown of its occurrence in different continents is 0.3 to 30.4% in Africa, 0.1 to 21.4% in Asia, 0.8 to 41.2% in Australia, 0 to 29.9% in Europe, 0.4 to 50.2% in North America and 0.5 to 50.5% in South America. More specific estimates for its prevalence in certain areas are 2% in Germany, 43% in Brazil, 35% in Nicaragua, more than 80% in certain areas of Africa and 83% in Cote d'Ivoire.

Endolimax is not considered to be a pathogen but simply colonizes and is noninvasive in the large intestines (colon). The presence of *Endolimax nana* trophozoites or cysts indicate fecal contamination of food or water or children eating feces. Immature cysts pass in feces into the environment. The immature cysts will undergo maturation and be ingested, passing through the stomach into the small intestines. At that point they excyst and a trophozoite is released.

The trophozoite will pass into the large intestines and reproduce producing additional trophozoites and cysts. Trophozoites and immature cysts may be passed in the feces into the environment. Trophozoites rapidly die outside the host. However, cysts are resistant and may survive for days up to weeks in the environment. When trophozoites and cysts are ingested, trophozoites are rapidly killed by the gastric juices in the stomach. The cysts will pass into the large intestines and release trophozoites completing the lifecycle. Trophozoites may survive in the colon for more than 17 years.

The clinical significance of *Endolimax nana* is unknown. Cumulative information suggests that *Endolimax* does not cause illness. However, there are reports it will cause abdominal pain, diarrhea and weight loss.

The diarrhea may be intermittent or chronic. These symptoms may not be due to *Endolimax nana* but the result of co-infection with other parasites.

Endolimax nana is diagnosed through microscopic evaluation of stool showing trophozoites and/or cysts. A PCR test would show *Endolimax* DNA. Serological blood testing may be positive for both *Endolimax* IgG and IgM antibodies. The presence of IgG antibody may only signify a previous or old infection. Positive IgM antibody would indicate an ongoing or recent infection.

No treatment is indicated for most infections of *Endolimax nana*. If treatment is initiated because of the ongoing symptoms, Metronidazole is the preferred first line choice. It would be given 250 mg three times a day for 7 to 10 days or 35 to 50 mg/kg/da for 7 to 10 days.

Prevention is through proper hygiene, use of clean drinking water, properly preparing foods and avoiding fecal contamination. Before eating, all fresh vegetables or fruits should be fwashed with clean water. Drinking water from deep wells is more likely to be contaminated with *Endolimax* and should be boiled before use. The presence of *Endolimax nana* in stool is a red flag that other pathogenic parasites may also be present.

Espundia. Kala Azar

Leishmania
Leishmaniasis:
Leishmania braziliensis. Leishmania tropica.
  Leishmania donovani
Cutaneous Leishmaniasis
Mucocutaneous Leishmaniasis
Visceral Leishmaniasis

Leishmania protozoa are found on every continent in the world except Antarctica and Australia. Estimates are that worldwide there are 12 million infected people in 88 different countries, 16 developed and 72 developing countries. It has now spread to non-endemic areas. Each year there are about 2 million new cases of leishmaniasis with 70,000 deaths due to complications from delayed or inadequate treatment. Leishmaniasis primarily occurs, is endemic, in Ethiopia, India, the Sudan, Bangladesh, the Middle East, Asia, Tropics, North Africa, Southern Europe especially Turkey and Central and South America but not in Uruguay or Chile. 90% of cases of leishmaniasis occur in Iran, Afghanistan, Syria, Saudi Arabia, Brazil and Peru. Those that reside or are travelers for business, adventure, recreation or military personnel deployed to these areas are at risk of acquiring leishmaniasis. Missionaries, construction workers, Peace Corps volunteers or others through outdoor activities like agricultural workers, hunting, fishing or mining and especially outdoors at twilight or night in endemic areas are at risk to acquire leishmaniasis.

Even though there are as many as 20 types of *Leishmania* that may infect people, most infections are the result of three primary types or species, *Leishmania tropica*, *Leishmania braziliensis* and *Leishmania donovani*. Different species are found in different parts of the world and will produce different patterns of clinical illness, cutaneous leishmaniasis, mucocutaneous leishmaniasis and visceral leishmaniasis. The incubation, time between initiation of infection and onset of illness varies depending upon the host immunity and species producing infection. There is also a distinction between Old World (*Leishmania tropica, Leishmania donovani*) and New World species (*Leishmania viannia braziliensis, Leishmania chagasi, Leishmania mexicana*) producing disease patterns and variable response to treatment measures. New World refers to land discoveries by the early explorers versus the Old World, areas of the world known before exploration occurred.

The illness is transmitted by the bite of an infected female sandfly. Sandflies become infected during a blood feeding on infected people, dogs, rodents and other mammalian wild and natural reservoir hosts. Their blood has a cell type called a macrophage that is infected with the amastigote *Leishmania* stage. The macrophage will release the amastigote into the bloodstream. After a blood meal, in the sandfly gut the amastigote undergoes development into the mobile flagellated stage, the promastigote. The flagella is a whiplike projection that allows movement of the promastigote.

The promastigote moves and migrates to the sandfly's feeding apparatus, the proboscis. When an infected sandfly bites and feeds, it injects promastigotes into the skin and bloodstream. Macrophages in the skin and bloodstream will ingest the promastigotes. Promastigotes may also enter dendritic cells, special immune system cells found in the skin and body tissues. The macrophage's function is to ingest and digest germs of all types. However, inside the macrophage the promastigote evades and escapes destruction and will transform into the amastigote stage. It will block certain immune system products and trigger others that turn off the body's immune system allowing progression of disease. The infected macrophage will rupture and release amastigotes. These amastigotes will infect additional macrophages and other phagocytic cells.

Diagnosis Depends on Testing but also Exposure Risk and a High Index of Suspicion of Disease

History of travel or residence in an endemic area where there is a predominant specific type of *Leishmania* species.

Presence of skin lesions on exposed areas of the face, neck or limbs.

Microscopic visualization of amastigotes from a skin scraping biopsy or culture. A culture requires a special medium and may take a week or longer for results.

Skin antigen testing, Montenegro test may be falsely negative in those with an impaired immune system. It may not become positive for up to three months after infection started.

Serology, blood or urine tests showing antibodies or measuring antigen specific for *Leishmania*. It may not differentiate between new, old or relapsing infection.

Molecular, PCR testing on a lesion or blood sample measuring *Leishmania* DNA. PCR testing is the new gold standard and the most accurate and reliable test. This technology may not be accessible in different parts of the world.

Cutaneous skin disease has a large number of parasites recoverable at the skin lesion site, but low antibody production with little immune system response. Relapsing or mucocutaneous leishmaniasis has few parasites at the site of disease but a robust immune system response with high levels of antibodies produced.

Treatment depends on a number of factors: Is it a new or relapsing infection, the aggressiveness and risk of disseminating or progressing to mucosal involvement of the specific *Leishmania* species producing the illness, its susceptibility and resistance to therapeutic agents, availability of the different therapeutic agents and the overall health status and host immune system factors and function. Relapse means persistence of the intracellular stage versus new or reinfection. It may be hard to distinguish between these. Co-infection, especially with HIV reduces treatment efficacy and clinical response as well as increases the rate of relapses. Generally, relapses are more difficult to treat than a primary infection.

Cutaneous Leishmaniasis

Cutaneous leishmaniasis is most likely to occur in Brazil, Peru, Syria, Saudi Arabia, Iran and Afghanistan. In America, cases may occur in Texas and Oklahoma. It is the most common type of leishmaniasis and most often due to *Leishmania braziliensis*. *Leishmania braziliensis* is reported to have 700,000 to 1.2 million new cases and 50,000 deaths each year. One or more localized skin sores may develop weeks to months after an infected sandfly bite. Infection of the macrophages in the skin causes superficial skin sores and cutaneous disease. When infection is due to Old World species, lesions start with painless bumps that develop into a cyst that most often will heal on its own over 1 to 2 years. New World strains start with a painless bump that develops into a hard knot or nodule that will become a painful ulcer.

Ulcers may become infected with bacteria. *Leishmania mexicana* New World infections may heal in 3 to 6 months. *Leishmania braziliensis* sores may take longer to heal spontaneously.

Infection may spread to other organs like the lining of the nose producing nasal lesions. Cutaneous infection may however produce little or no additional symptoms. They may remain asymptomatic and heal spontaneously as evidenced by scars on those living in endemic areas. However, it may result in disfigurement or scarring with deformity depending upon the infecting species.

A healed bite site may be a nodule most often occurring after *Leishmania tropica* infection in the old world and *Leishmania mexicana* and *braziliensis* as the new world species. There may be 1 to 10 skin lesions most commonly seen on the exposed body areas, face, neck and extremities. Each site may represent a single infected sandfly biting repetitively or each may be the result of different infected sandflies bites.

Cutaneous disease may progress and spread to distant skin areas (disseminated cutaneous leishmaniasis) and affect two or more and sometimes as many as 10 non-adjacent skin areas of the body. There may be more than 10 and up to thousands of bumpy ulcerated sores that develop. This spread of disease is not common in children. It is more likely to occur in individuals with a compromised or deficient immune system. These are different from single skin lesions with sores in different forms, papules (bumps), nodules and ulcers. This type of disease is more likely with one type of *Leishmania*, *Leishmania braziliensis* producing ulcers or *Leishmania tropica* which is more likely to produce papules, plaques and combination lesions.

In another type of skin infection called diffuse cutaneous leishmaniasis there may be multiple nodules or ulcers or mucosal (moist lining of the mouth or nose) involvement in exposed body areas. It is also not likely to occur in children. It is most likely to occur from *Leishmania mexicana* and *Leishmania viannia braziliensis* infection and those with impaired immunity. They may have a deficiency in their T lymphocyte function that allows lesion extension. Overall, it responds poorly to treatment but when medicine is combined with immunotherapy it has a 50% cure rate and long remission time.

There may be relapses (Leishmaniasis recidivans) years and decades after skin disease occurring at the site of the initial healed lesion. This may occur whether they were treated or untreated. It is most likely due to *Leishmania tropica*.

Leishmania tropica and Leishmania donovani may be spread from one person to another through contaminated blood transfusions, bone marrow and solid organ transplants, needlestick injuries and from an infected pregnant person to her unborn child.

Mucocutaneous Leishmaniasis

Mucocutaneous leishmaniasis is also known as "Espundia". It is more likely to occur in Bolivia, Costa Rica, Afghanistan, Brazil, Colombia, Paraguay, Ecuador, Venezuela and Turkey. New world species are more likely to progress to the moist lining of the mouth or nose. If the host has a weakened or partial immune system deficiency or compromised by illness, organ transplant or by co-infection especially with HIV, there may be uncontrolled disseminated or diffuse skin and mucous membranes spread. This occurs through the body by macrophages in the bloodstream or lymphatic system. It is the most destructive of all skin leishmaniasis spreading to deeper layers than the lining surfaces producing mucocutaneous disease. It may occur at the same time of cutaneous infection or be delayed by months or years. Early detection and treatment lower the risk of mucocutaneous disease.

Mucocutaneous disease may Involve the nose, throat, eyelids, face, larynx, lips, inside cheeks and roof of mouth. It may start with itching then crusting of the nose and nasal bleeding. It may cause obstruction and destruction of mouth and nasal tissue resulting in disfigurement. It may cause difficulty breathing as well as eating problems causing malnutrition. It is more likely to occur with Leishmania viannia braziliensis. Depending upon the specific species of Leishmania causing the infection, there may be a poor response to treatment requiring a longer course of therapy.

Visceral Leishmaniasis

Visceral leishmaniasis is also known as Kala azar, Black fever or Dumdum fever. It is caused by Leishmania donovani and Leishmania infantum. It has a worldwide distribution with as many as 206,000 to 500,000 new cases each year. New cases occur in clusters with more than 90% reported in India, Nepal, Ethiopia, Sudan, Bangladesh and Brazil. Unfortunately, in these areas, care is often unavailable or inadequate.

Like other forms of leishmaniasis, it is spread by the bite of the infected female sandfly. It is a multisystem multiorgan disease.

Infection occurs in the internal organs, most often the spleen, liver and bone marrow. Symptoms are an enlarged spleen, irregular recurring fever, low white blood cell count, anemia, weight loss and weakness. These symptoms may occur weeks to months, often 2 to 8 months, after the bite of the infected sandfly.

Those with immune system problems, immunosuppression or immunocompromise, especially those co-infected with HIV have more severe lesions, poorer treatment response and increased occurrence of relapses. In some areas there is a 20 to 40% co-infection rate with HIV. If visceral leishmaniasis is untreated, it is nearly uniformly fatal in 2 to 3 years with a 95% death rate. Death is from just wasting away or from acquiring other infections that in their weakened state prove to be fatal. Kala-azar is second only to malaria in causing deaths from a parasitic infection. Those untreated also serve as a reservoir to spread infection to other susceptible individuals through sandfly feeding.

Treatment

Treatment is species and clinical disease specific. Overall, for cutaneous leishmaniasis, if the individual is not immunosuppressed, then simply monitor and allow the lesion to heal on its own. Depending upon the specific species it may take months to years for the lesion to heal. Signs of healing began with flattening and decreased size of the skin lesion. For those effectively treated there would be at least a 50% reduction after treatment was started. For all types of leishmaniasis, treatment would include anti-*Leishmania* medication given as a shot in the muscle or into the bloodstream, taken orally or topically. If there is an immunodeficiency, a risk of developing disseminated or mucosal disease, the lesion is large (more than 5 cm, more than 2 inches), multiple lesions or located at a site that is likely to produce disfigurement (on the face, ears or near joints), then consider active treatment. As long as a person has active lesions, they serve as a source of infection spread through sandfly feeding. Treating reduces the pool of infected people that serves as a source of infection spread.

The species may be quickly and accurately identified as discussed with the polymerase chain reaction (PCR) test to allow selection of the most effective treatment approach. The World Health Organization, WHO, keeps an inventory of best treatment options for specific *Leishmania* species based on susceptibility and resistance patterns.

For treatment options selection of a specific medication for topical, parenteral or oral administration will be determined by the specific species of *Leishmania* producing the illness and its response and susceptibility pattern to different medications. Medication given through an IV or as a shot requires the child to be treated and followed either through a clinic or admitted to a hospital for care and observation. More severe disease requires more aggressive therapy at a higher care level center. These individuals have poorer compliance because these facilities are not available or simply too far to utilize. For cutaneous Leishmaniasis, medicine may be directly applied or injected into a skin lesion. Topical treatment would be preferred for uncomplicated skin disease when there are only a few lesions and there is minimal risk of disease spread or progression.

Topical medications would be Paromomycin (is cheap and may be used in outpatient therapy), Imiquimod and Antimony injected into the skin lesions. Injected Antimony is not used for the *Leishmania viannia braziliensis* subgenus due to a risk of spread of disease. These measures are painful and may result in scarring. Topical treatment with Paromomycin or Methylbenzethonium would be twice a day for 20 days. Alternatively skin lesions may be treated by using a probe with different temperatures singly or in combination with other therapies. Very cold temperature (cryotherapy) or very warm temperature (thermotherapy) have been used with success. Cryotherapy would be −319°F every 3 to 7 days for 1 to 5 sessions. Cryotherapy has been found to be very effective in producing complete remission for cutaneous disease when combined with other topical treatment measures. Alternatively, thermotherapy would be 1 to 2 sessions with 122°F for 30 seconds and is also very effective when combined with other therapies against *Leishmania mexicana*.

Oral medications that could be used if topical treatment fails, relapses occur or mucocutaneous or visceral disease develops are Miltefosine, Ketoconazole and Fluconazole. Intravenous treatment would be with Pentavalent Antimony, liposomal Amphotericin B or Pentamidine Isethionate. More aggressive treatment options are required for individuals that are immunocompromised or at risk of disseminated disease due to the specific *Leishmania* species producing infection. Fluconazole is dosed at 200 mg/day for six weeks, Ketoconazole 600 mg/day for 28 days or Miltefosine 2.5 mg/kg/da for 28 days. Pentavalent Antimonial would be given 15–20 mg/kg/day intramuscular or intravenous for 10 to 20 days and liposomal Amphotericin B given IV for 25 to 30 days. For those with co-infection, liposomal Amphotericin B is the treatment of choice. Pentoxifylline (400 mg given 3 times a day) could be added to

10 to 20 days treatment with Pentavalent Antimonial. Unfortunately, each of these would require treatment to be received at a clinic.

Miltefosine now appears to be the preferred product for treatment of New and Old-World species cutaneous disease. It kills both amastigote and promastigote stages. It reduces the time for the ulcer to heal and reduces spread. It is well tolerated taken orally with few side effects. It Has a 68 to 83% cure rate for cutaneous Leishmaniasis. It is given usually at 1.8–2.5 mg/kg/day for 28 days. However, when used to treat diffuse cutaneous Leishmaniasis, relapses may occur. Alternatively, some data reported Meglumine Antimonate to be more effective for old world species than Miltefosine for the treatment of cutaneous Leishmaniasis. It may be given to children as an intramuscular shot at 20 mg/kg/day for 20 days and requires a higher-level care center. Its cure rate may be 45 to 53%. For children younger than five years of age the cure rate may be less than 25%.

Overall cure rates vary between 17 and 69%. Infection with New World species may respond better to the combination of liposomal Amphotericin B and Antimonial products (Meglumine and Pentavalent). The efficacy for New World leishmaniasis is 25% for those younger than 5 years of age and 75% for those 5 to 14 years of age. For Old World leishmaniasis, Sodium Stibogluconate (SSG) and liposomal Amphotericin B may be the treatments of choice. There is a 35% cure rate for those 15 years of age or younger and 72% cure rate when intralesional treatment is used for those 13 years of age and younger. When combined with cryotherapy for those 13 years of age and younger, the cure rate is 41%. Sodium Stibogluconate has a 95% cure rate for visceral leishmaniasis. Interferon gamma has been given singly or combined with the Tuberculosis vaccine BCG. The BCG vaccination may be given along with heat killed *Leishmania mexicana* promastigotes. With the different treatments, the cure rate for *Leishmania braziliensis* may be 25 to 85%

Children respond less well to treatment and have a higher rate of initial treatment failure and relapses. The younger the child the poorer the response to treatment. Recommendations for treatment of leishmaniasis in adults may not be extrapolated to accurately and effectively treat children. Children have different pharmacokinetics, metabolic processing of these agents compared to adults reaching lower medicine levels and maintaining a shorter period for the medicine to be effective. In addition to age, the shorter time between onset of illness and initiation of treatment diminishes the therapeutic response.

Compared to adults, children are diagnosed at an earlier stage. There seems to be less time for an effective immune system response to be activated.

It appears an effective immune system response plus medication combination is required to produce the best therapeutic clinical response. Treatment started before 8 weeks of infection onset is less effective due to low levels of interferon and high levels of interleukin 10 causing an inadequate host immune response and blocked parasite elimination. Children with cutaneous Leishmaniasis and visceral Leishmaniasis may be effectively treated with a combination of liposomal Amphotericin B and Miltefosine.

As a general rule, all forms of leishmaniasis should be reevaluated 26 weeks after the last treatment was administered. For cutaneous and muco-cutaneous leishmaniasis, monitor skin lesions for 6 to 12 months after the final treatment for evidence of treatment success and persistence or relapse of skin lesions. Monitor all cutaneous lesions for secondary bacterial infections.

Preventive measures are to avoid sandfly exposure by reducing outdoor activities from dusk until dawn in endemic areas. Protect and cover exposed skin areas with long pants, long sleeve shirts, apply a Permethrin based insect repellent directly to the face, neck, hands, other exposed skin areas and clothing. Protect pets from sandfly exposure or biting. Sleep in areas that have air-conditioning or are screened or use beds covered with nets treated with Permethrin.

"Cured" patients are unlikely to become reinfected with the same species. After recovering they are less susceptible and may develop lifelong immunity for the specific infecting species. However, because of multiple *Leishmania* species, additional infections are possible with different exposures. Several candidate vaccinations have been in clinical trials but to date none have been effective for general use. Insect spraying programs have been implemented to reduce the sandfly population.

Giardia

Giardiasis
Giardia duodenalis, Giardia intestinalis, Giardia lamblia

Giardia is one of the most prevalent intestinal parasitic protozoan infections and the most common cause of infectious diarrhea in the world. Estimates are it has a prevalence of 2 to 5% in the developed world and 20 to 30% in developing countries. 20–40% of those living with poor sanitation or limited access to safe, treated drinking water will have antibodies to *Giardia* showing current or previous infection. Annually more than 280 million new cases occur globally with 2.5 million deaths due to *Giardia* diarrhea disease. In the United States there are an estimated 1.2 million cases each year with regional differences and more cases found in the Northeast. Eight different genetic subtypes of *Giardia* have been identified.

It exists in two stages, the environmental resistant cyst stage and actively moving trophozoites in the intestinal tract. It is transmitted by direct oral ingestion of infective cysts. It may be waterborne through ingestion of contaminated or untreated drinking water when hiking, camping, swimming or enjoying recreational water activities at water parks, hot tubs, swimming pools, spa, lakes, creeks, streams and ponds or spread from person to person. Private wells could be a source because they are not required to have testing or water treatment.

Cysts may be spread through undercooked, contaminated food or unwashed produce, raw vegetables or fruit. Irrigation and fertilization measures with human fecal waste, food processing and packing especially if done with unwashed hands may be sources of contamination. International travelers and internationally adopted children may acquire *Giardia* when visiting or living in endemic areas with poor sanitation. Internationally adopted children may be infested with more than one type of parasite.

Giardia has a high prevalence in children less than four years of age. They may still be in diapers, have minimal or no toilet skills and attend a day care center. Also, those working at day care centers have a higher risk of acquiring *Giardia*. Clustering of *Giardia* outbreaks may occur in family members and childcare providers from infected children. In these situations, they may be crowded together which also promotes the spread of *Giardia*. Household pets may be infected and serve as a source of giardiasis spread.

Giardia will cycle among numerous mammals. Its cysts are highly infectious when passed in the stool and it takes only 10 to 25 cysts ingested to successfully colonize the small intestines. The duodenum is the most common site where the environment and host factors are most favorable. The ileum and jejunum, middle and last segments of the small intestine are less likely to be colonized. In the intestines, trophozoites are released from cysts. They may remain free and multiply in the intestines or may attach and penetrate the intestinal lining. From there they may spread to other organs. Trophozoites that pass into the colon (large intestine) may transform back into cysts. Both cysts and trophozoites may be seen in the stool. Once they are ingested, varying degrees of illness may follow with some individuals having no symptoms while others have mild self-limited, moderate or even severe symptoms. There are reports that *Giardia* colonization may have a protective role reducing the occurrence of diarrhea from other infectious causes. It may out compete other germs for necessary nutrients.

Most cases of giardiasis occur in healthy individuals with a normal immune system. For these individuals, infection is most likely asymptomatic or self-limited. They may have spontaneous recovery within weeks following ingestion of the cysts. This is especially true for children who have a higher rate of asymptomatic infections. It is possible to have protracted or intermittent shedding of cysts even for those who are asymptomatic or have mild symptoms. Estimates are one individual may over months shed between 10 million and up to 100 million cysts in their stool each day. Cysts are hardy and may survive in water and food or on surfaces for weeks up to several months. They are resistant to chlorine and other disinfecting agents.

The incubation, time between acquisition of infection and onset of symptoms is usually within two weeks, on average around eight days. Stools may have a distinctive foul-smelling sulfur, struck match or discharged fireworks smell. Symptoms may include large volume, watery diarrhea which is the most common symptom, abdominal pain worsened by eating, bloating, nausea, vomiting, fever, loss of appetite, weight loss and fatty stools due to malabsorption of nutrients. Weight loss due to malabsorption is more likely to occur with chronic infection. Chronic and more severe infections are more likely to occur in those with a compromised immune system either immunosuppressed or immunodeficient. For these individuals *Giardia* may invade deeper tissue layers and spread to sites outside the intestinal tract. These individuals are more likely to also have influenza-like symptoms with sweating and body aches.

Malabsorption results from damage to the lining of the intestinal tract and will lead to iron deficiency, fat and water-soluble vitamin deficiencies and intestinal bacterial and yeast overgrowth. The trophozoites compete with the body for nutrients and also by attaching to the intestinal lining produce a mechanical block preventing absorption of nutrients. Through activation of the body's immune system, it may trigger other illnesses like asthma, chronic fatigue, hives, joint pain, reactive arthritis, irritable bowel syndrome and uveitis. Hives may be acute, become chronic and occur from pressure on the skin.

The gold standard for diagnosis of giardiasis is microscopically identifying *Giardia* protozoan trophozoites or cysts in a stool sample. The accuracy of this test is dependent upon the numbers of parasites being excreted in the stool and also a high degree of luck in visualizing them. A molecular test, PCR identifying *Giardia* DNA or microRNA segments is much more accurate in demonstrating ongoing infection. Serology tests measuring IgG antibodies in the blood are not specific for ongoing infection but indicate at some point infection did occur. If IgM antibodies are detected this would be more consistent with an ongoing or recent *Giardia* infection.

Diagnosis may also be made through evaluation of small bowel biopsies of the duodenum or terminal ileum which may show both inflammatory changes and *Giardia* trophozoites in the intestinal epithelial lining. The terminal ileum may have a greater number of trophozoites present. Trophozoites may be observed either attached to or in the host epithelial lining cells.

The goals for care are to maintain hydration and prevent dehydration, shorten how long diarrhea persists and reduce the severity of other symptoms. Giardiasis may be self-limited and resolve without treatment in 3 to 6 weeks. For those who are symptomatic, focus on preventing complications and reduce the risk of spread. Maintain hydration with one half strength Gatorade, mixed half-and-half with water. This is an excellent liquid to maintain hydration. If diarrhea is severe, undiluted Gatorade may be preferred for its higher electrolyte concentration. Avoid milk and dairy products.

These will worsen cramps and diarrhea due to a relative lactose intolerance. Alternatively, popsicles and Jello are primarily water and usually well tolerated.

Metronidazole is the medicine of choice to treat *Giardia* infections. Treatment is generally very successful with a success rate of 80 to 95% with a standard oral dose of 15 mg/kg/day divided into three equal doses given for 5 to 7 days or as a one-time dose. The maximum for each dose is 250 mg. If diarrhea continues or reoccurs, there may be persistent/refractory infection with treatment failure. For treatment failures, retreat at a higher dose of 40–45 mg/kg with doses divided every eight hours for 10 days or use a combination of different medications. This will achieve another 10% treatment success.

Alternative medicines are available and have proven effective in treating giardiasis. Furazolidone is given orally and dosed 6–8 mg/kg/day divided into 3 or 4 equal doses for 7 to 10 days. Albendazole is also given orally and dosed 15 mg/kg as a single daily (maximum 400 mg) dose for 5 to 7 days. Nitazoxanide is given orally for 3 days and is dosed 100 mg twice a day for those 1 to 3 years of age, 200 mg twice a day for those 4 to 11 years of age and for those 12 years of age and older 500 mg twice a day. Tinidazole is given 50 mg/kg as a one-time dose, Secnidazole is given 30 mg/kg as a 1-time dose. Ornidazole is dosed 40–50 mg/kg as a 1-time dose. Those younger than two years of age seem to be an entirely different population in their response to medicine and are at the greatest risk of having treatment failure with any antiparasitic agent. This is most likely the result of how their system absorbs, processes and metabolizes the medicine with different absorption rates and gastric pH affecting drug metabolism. Eradication of the infection should be confirmed especially in children less than two years of age who have a higher rate of treatment failure and recurrences.

Every individual diagnosed with giardiasis should have a repeat microscopic stool examination and PCR done four weeks after treatment was completed. Estimates are that 8.3% of all Giardia infections continued to be refractory after two cycles of Metronidazole. Treatment failure may be due to noncompliance or altered absorption of the medicine due to gut inflammation. Quinine may be given as a second line drug for treatment failures and is dosed 6 mg/kg/day for five days. Estimates are that it is 100% effective treating giardiasis. It is unfortunately not approved for use in pediatric patients and is used "off label".

There is no vaccination for giardiasis. It is not killed by chlorine but removed by filtration. Bringing water to a boil will kill cysts.

Preventive measures include proper hygiene. good handwashing, observation of appropriate sanitation measures and proper disposal of fecal or contaminated materials. Wash all produce in clean water before consumption. Try to maintain good health by taking a daily probiotic. The best probiotics contain Lactobacillus and/or Bifidobacterium. Probiotics will reduce the length of the illness, minimize symptoms of infection and decrease the number of trophozoites that are produced and shed.

Guinea Worm

Dracunculus
Dracunculus medinensis. Dracunculiasis

Dracunculus is a round worm, nematode parasite. It traditionally occurs in remote, rural areas where there is limited or no access to safe drinking water or consumption of raw or undercooked fish or other aquatic animals containing water fleas infected with *Dracunculus* larvae It has been reported in areas of Asia and Sub-Saharan Africa. Estimates in the early 1980's were there were as many as 3.5 million people infected with Guinea worm. In some areas as many as 15 to 70% of the population had antibodies to *Dracunculus* indicating active, recent or past infection. As many as 20 Sub-Saharan countries had active disease but since 1986 when an educational program was put in place the number of cases has been reduced by 98%. Through the provision of safe drinking water, Pakistan, India, Senegal, Cameroon, Yemen and Kenya have eradicated the disease.

There were 55,000 cases reported worldwide in 2007. By 2016 Dracunculiasis had been limited to Chad, Mali, Ethiopia, Southern Sudan with some cases in Angola, Ghana and Nigeria. Cases may occur in non-endemic areas due to Peace Corps and other volunteers, travelers returning home and immigrants and refugees moving from an endemic area. More recently only a handful of cases were reported with 27 cases in 2020 from Angola, Ethiopia, Southern Sudan, Mali, Chad and Cameroon, 15 cases in 2021 and 13 cases in 2022.

There is a predictable seasonal pattern related to rainfall for the occurrence of Dracunculiasis. During the dry season for wet areas there are limited sources of drinking water, stagnant ponds, creeks, riverbeds, wells and cisterns all potentially harboring infected water fleas. Alternatively in dry areas transmission occurs during the rainy season when there are surface water sources available.

Infection begins with the oral ingestion of water contaminated with infected water fleas. The water fleas are killed by the stomach acidity releasing larvae. The larvae pass into the duodenum, the first segment of the small intestines where they penetrate the lining and wall. From there the larvae will pass into the connective tissue of the abdominal wall and chest. In 60 to 90 days after the infection started the larvae undergo two additional developmental stages and mature in the abdomen into male and female adults. At that point they mate and the male dies.

The female continues to develop over the next 10 to 14 months and migrates along bone and muscle planes to the surface of the body. The female may grow to around 1 meter, 39 inches in length and be 1 to 2 millimeters in width. A blister will form at the skin surface which will over three days fill with fluid and pop, leaving an ulcer. The skin lesion may occur anywhere but more than 90% are located on the legs with most below the knees. The female worm may migrate to the eyes, heart, lungs or spinal cord and at these sites produce pockets of infection, abscesses. An individual may have more than one worm with as many as two up to 40 worms and ulcers reported at the same time. The ulcer is uncomfortable producing burning pain and the individual for relief will submerge the area in water. The female will begin to push out from the ulcer. Water triggers the female worm to release a white substance containing a swarm of thousands of motile, immature, rhabditiform larvae into the water. These larvae will survive for only three days in the water. To continue their development, they will be ingested by the water fleas. In the water flea over a two-week period, they will go through two additional developmental stages. The lifecycle is completed when these infected water fleas are ingested by people. The diagnosis is made by observing the worms in the skin ulcers.

There will be no symptoms until just before the blister develops when the adult female worm reaches the subcutaneous tissue. As a result of activation of the immune system, there will be stinging and itching of the skin, fever, hives, shortness of breath, dizziness, nausea, vomiting and diarrhea. The ulcer will have a burning pain. It is possible for an infected individual to have pain for an additional 12 to 18 months after the worm has emerged. If the adult female worm ruptures or dies in the body, in muscle layers or subcutaneous skin, it will release larvae resulting in inflammation.

Dead worms may also calcify. There will be painful inflammation along the tract of a dead worm.

Humans were believed to be the only host for *Dracunculus*. However, it is now known that dogs in Chad, Ethiopia and Mali, domesticated and feral cats in Chad and Mali, baboons in Ethiopia all may likewise be infected with *Dracunculus*. It is unclear if they have always served as hosts for this parasite or if this has been a recent specific adaptation that has occurred in response to reducing its occurrence in people. In animals, *Dracunculus* will progress through the same developmental stages as in humans. There were 1000 cases reported in dogs in Chad in 2016. They may become infected by eating contaminated fish. These animal cases may account for the reemergence of human cases of Guinea worm in Ethiopia, Chad, Mali and Angola. There are an additional 100 "suspected" human cases reported.

There is no treatment for Guinea worm infections. Supportive care focuses on the care of the ulcer. Keeping a wet dressing or cover makes it less painful. Give ibuprofen or acetaminophen for pain. There is a high risk of a bacterial infection developing in the ulcer. Bacteria may cause a wound abscess, infected joints or spread throughout the body causing sepsis. Death from *Dracunculus* infection is rare but occurs at a rate of 1% from secondary bacterial infections. Keep the area clean and disinfected with an antiseptic like peroxide followed by an antibiotic ointment or cream to minimize bacterial infections. Adding a topical steroid may promote healing.

Metronidazole given orally 25 mg/kg/day divided into three equal doses for 10 days does not kill the worms but decreases inflammation from the worms. The definitive treatment is to unwind the worm around a matchstick or something else similar and then pull the worm with gentle traction advancing several centimeters every day. This is combined with the worm itself exiting the ulcer over 3 to 10 weeks. As a result, the worm is removed over several weeks to several months. Do not apply too much pressure because this may break the worm leaving part remaining within the skin. There is little or no immunity after infections. Recurrent infections will occur with repeated intake of contaminated water.

There is no effective vaccination for *Dracunculus*. Preventive measures center on education about the parasite, only consuming safe drinking water and stopping more parasites from being introduced into the water. Drinking water may be made safe by boiling or filtering it through special filters like a nylon or cloth filter, plastic or some other type of mesh filter. Identify those with active infection by skin sores and keep them from submerging the involved skin in surface drinking water. Obtain drinking water from a safe deep well source. Treat surface waters that may have water fleas with an insecticide, "Abate" and larvicide, "Tempo" which kills the larvae but is safe for human consumption. With a reemergence of cases of Dracunculiasis and armed with information about additional animal reservoirs, ongoing, constant surveillance and education are critical to continue and eliminate future *Dracunculus* disease.

Heterophyes. Metagonimus

Heterophyiasis
Heterophyes heterophyes
Metagonimus yokogawai

Heterophyiasis is an infection with the intestinal flukes *Heterophyes* and *Metagonimus*. There are at least 29 types of the *Heterophyes* fluke causing infection in people. Estimates are that there are more than 7 million people worldwide infected with heterophyiasis. The most common types are *Heterophyes heterophyes* and *Metagonimus yokogawai*. It has a complex lifecycle in mammals (people, dogs, foxes and cats), aquatic birds like heron, snails and fish. Several families of fish may be infected, tilapia, perch, gobies, mullet, fountain darter and shrimp. It has a wide distribution occurring naturally in Japan, Lao Peoples Democratic Republic, China, Taiwan, the Philippines, Korea, Thailand, India, Nepal, Sudan, Sri Lanka, Serbia, Manchuria, the Nile Delta area, Tunisia, Iran, Israel, Turkey, Spain, the Balkans, parts of the old Soviet Union, Mexico, Texas and Hawaii. It may occur in other parts of the world from imported infected fish. Children may become infected by ingestion of infected raw, smoked, salted, marinated, undercooked snakes, snails, frogs, clams and fish.

The prevalence is seasonal with the highest rate occurring in the summer and spring and lowest in the winter. This correlates with environmental factors for the snail population. Estimates are that between 22 and 42% of all tilapia fish are infected with *Heterophyes*. Similarly, prevalence rates for infection will vary with 13 to 33.8% of people in parts of Egypt being infected with *Heterophyes*, 1.2 to 42.9% of those in Korea and now 100 percent of those in Vietnam reported being infected with *Heterophyes*. Variations are related to differences in food habits and rate of local fish infection.

Adult worms in the intestinal tract of mammals and aquatic birds will produce and release eggs into the feces which then pass into water. In brackish and freshwater rivers, lakes and creeks, the eggs hatch into the miracidium which will penetrate snails. In the snails the miracidium develops into the cercariae. Cercariae will then pass into the water from the snail and infect fish. In the fish the cercariae will produce a shell-like case (cyst) under the scales, in muscle or skin and form the metacercaria which are infectious. When aquatic birds and mammals ingest the infected fish, the metacercaria in about four hours will be released (excyst) in the small intestines. Juvenile flukes will then penetrate the intestinal lining into the intestinal wall. There in 5 to 10 days they develop into adults which may remain stuck in the intestinal wall or migrate to and become attached to the mucosal lining of the small intestines.

Adult worms are very small, approximately 2 mm in length. They feed on the host's intestinal tissue. In around nine days, adults will begin to produce and release eggs. One adult worm may produce only 35 to 45 eggs a day. The adults stuck in the intestinal wall may have their eggs pass through the lymphatics or bloodstream to distant organs including the heart, brain, spinal cord, lungs, liver and spleen. In the different organs they induce the body's inflammatory response producing a granuloma and scar tissue. Otherwise for those adults attached to the mucosal lining, their eggs are released and pass in the feces back into the environment.

Mild infections with few worms may produce no symptoms. Heavier infections with a large number of worms may produce irritable bowel like symptoms with colicky abdominal pain, heartburn, loss of appetite, nausea, malabsorption, weight loss, vomiting and diarrhea with mucus. Anemia may develop with intestinal ulcers and perforation. These symptoms may last for only one month even though the flukes may persist for 2 to 4 months up to one year in the gastrointestinal tract. With additional infections, symptoms may recur. Eggs that are passed to the cardiac muscle will produce heart damage with myocarditis, irregular heart rhythm, heart enlargement and potentially heart failure. Those passing to the brain and spinal cord may produce loss of sensation and movement function with weakness. Eggs may pass into the lungs and cause cough, shortness of breath and lung scarring. Eggs in the liver and spleen may cause fatigue, swelling of the abdomen, legs and feet.

The definitive diagnosis is made by microscopically observing eggs or adult worms in the feces. Adult worms are more likely to be seen in feces after treatment has been completed. Eggs may be unlikely to be visualized microscopically because adults produce only a limited number of eggs per day.

A blood test may show a high number of eosinophils. Serology tests measuring IgG antibody would show that an infection has occurred but may not specify an ongoing acute infection. The PCR test is more accurate and specific. It would show parasite DNA in the feces. Alternatively, a duodenal sample and biopsy may be collected by endoscopy.

Effective treatment for *Heterophyes* is with Praziquantel 10 to 25 mg/kg one time dose or alternatively 75 mg/kg divided into three equal doses given during a single day. *Metagonimus* would be treated with 25 mg/kg of Praziquantel 3 times a day for 1 day. The cure rate is 100%.

There is no vaccination for *Heterophyes*. Preventive measures include control of the snail population, appropriate sanitation and education about proper preparation of fish with effective cooking and not consuming raw, pickled, partially salted, marinated or undercooked fish especially imported from endemic areas. Wash hands and all cooking utensils used when preparing raw fish.

Hookworm

Necator americanus
Ancylostoma duodenale
Ancylostoma ceylanicum
Ancylostoma braziliense

Hookworms are soil transmitted helminths caused by the nematodes *Necator americanus*, *Ancylostoma duodenale* and *Ancylostoma ceylanicum*. They are acquired by larvae in contaminated soil contacting exposed skin areas. Estimates are now there are 1 billion people worldwide infected with hookworm causing 65,000 deaths a year. Infection and deaths occur mainly in tropic and subtropical areas. Residents of these areas and those doing missionary work in areas of poverty or poor hygiene are likely to acquire hookworm infection.

Vacationers to different Caribbean resorts are also at risk of acquiring hookworm infection. Refugees and adopted children from Southeast Asia are often infected with hookworm. The world's coastal areas have the highest rate of transmission because they have the optimal temperatures, humidity and sandy soil to promote survival of hookworm larvae. It is estimated that in China alone, 190 million people are infected with hookworm.

Necator americanus is the most common hookworm worldwide. It was considered the "New World" hookworm because of its area of distribution. *Ancylostoma duodenale* has likewise been viewed as the "Old World" hookworm. It may survive harsher environmental conditions. However, even though initially each had a more limited geographical range, both may now be spreading worldwide. *Ancylostoma ceylanicum* is the predominant hookworm of dogs and cats but it may be passed to humans.

Hookworm infections are found in residents of South and Southern China, Vietnam, South Africa, Southern India, Bangladesh, Sri Lanka, Sub-Saharan Africa, Egypt, Northern Australia, Central and South America,

Northern Argentina, Paraguay, Peru, El Salvador, Honduras, Germany, Austria, Belgium, Russia, the Caribbean area and the Pacific islands. It was thought to have been eradicated in the United States, but surveillance serology data shows it may never have gone away.

Infection begins with exposure of exposed skin to the L3 filariform infective larvae living in the soil. With the right environmental conditions, the L3 larvae may live in the soil for 3 to 4 weeks until it depletes its nutritional reserves. The larvae do not survive drying out. It will climb up a blade of grass and sway to increase chances of contact with skin. It will penetrate the skin or alternatively for *Ancylostoma duodenale* it may be taken into and penetrate the lining of the mouth.

The filariform L3 larvae becomes activated when it enters through pores, hair follicles or penetrates the skin. It travels through the blood vessels to the right side of the heart then passes into the blood vessels in the lungs. It breaks out of the lung blood vessels into the air exchange spaces. It will climb and be coughed up out of the bronchial tubes into the mouth and then swallowed back into the gastrointestinal tract. There the larvae go through 2 additional stages of development and become the adult worm. It takes around 5 to 8 weeks from the time the L3 larvae stage penetrates the skin until the worms have become mature adults in the small intestine.

The adults attach to the lining of the intestinal wall, feed on both blood and tissue. Blood delivers protein, iron and other nutrients for the hookworm. Adult worms mate and produce eggs. A female *Necator americanus* worm will produce 9,000 up to 10,000 eggs per day and live in the jejunum for up to 7 years. *Ancylostoma duodenale* females may produce 25,000 up to 30,000 eggs per day and likewise live for up to 7 years in the jejunum.

The eggs are passed with feces into the soil and in 24 to 48 hours with the proper moisture and shade, hatch into the L1 rhabditiform larval stage. The L1 larval stage feeds on bacteria and organic material in the soil and goes through 2 stages of development forming the infective L3 larval stage. *Ancylostoma duodenale* larvae may remain dormant in host muscle during the hottest and driest months of the year. They will sense an oncoming monsoon season and resume development to mature adults producing eggs. The eggs are more likely to survive in favorable environmental conditions.

Children 5 to 15 years of age have the greatest risk of acquiring hookworm infection because of exposure of both skin and contact with the contaminated soil. Children may acquire hookworm infection from playing on the ground. Walking barefoot is a prime way to acquire hookworm infection. In different parts of the world, human feces are used as fertilizer. The feces may be contaminated with hookworm eggs that have developed into the infective filariform larvae. This places those individuals working with crops at risk of acquiring infection through exposed skin on either hands or feet. Wearing gloves and shoes reduces the risk of hookworm infection. Effectively washing hands that may handle food, washing fresh produce and utensils used to prepare food reduces the risk of hookworm infection.

When the L3 larvae penetrate the skin, it will cause inflammation resulting in at times intense itching and burning called "ground itch". Generally, 10 days after skin penetration has occurred pulmonary symptoms including coughing and wheezing, shortness of breath, sore throat and fever may develop. These symptoms may last for one month. On occasion with hookworm infection there will be a bumpy rash on the buttocks.

Most infections are asymptomatic; however, the degree or number of symptoms are directly related to the number of infecting hookworms. As adults develop in the gastrointestinal tract, there may be abdominal pain, loss of appetite, gas, nausea, and diarrhea. These symptoms most likely occur 30 to 45 days after the skin infection. If *Ancylostoma* has been acquired by oral ingestion, the L3 larvae will penetrate the lining of the mouth. Symptoms that may occur would be nausea, vomiting, hoarseness, cough and sore throat. This is called "Wakana syndrome".

Heavy infections involving a large number of adults in the small intestines may result in iron deficiency anemia. *Ancylostoma duodenale* causes more blood loss with each adult worm consuming 0.15 ml of blood a day. The *Necator americanus* adult worm will consume 0.03 ml of blood a day. However heavy worm loads will cause significant blood loss over time. Children, women of childbearing potential/pregnant or those malnourished are vulnerable for the development of iron deficiency anemia.

Symptoms of iron deficiency anemia would include shortness of breath with activity, pallor or paleness and fatigue. Children may overall have slowed or no growth, impaired/damaged brain and intellectual development especially problems with memory, reasoning ability, reading comprehension and delayed motor (control of body movement, coordination and strength) development due to iron deficiency anemia. Additionally, from the parasite feeding, the body may have low protein causing distended abdomen, pot belly and swelling of the face and lower extremities.

Children may develop a rash called cutaneous larva migrans. This is the result of their contact with the infective larval stage of the dog hookworm

Ancylostoma braziliense. This larval stage has limited skin penetration. It remains in the outer layers of the skin causing a creeping elevated track that shows the movement and migration of the larvae. In the United States cutaneous larva migrans occurs in Florida and Gulf residents and vacationers to essentially any sandy beach.

Diagnosis of hookworm infection is based upon microscopic identification of eggs in feces. Serological tests may be used to measure IgG antibodies consistent with an infection occurring at some point in time. The presence of IgM antibodies would indicate a current or recent infection. A PCR test on feces would show hookworm DNA and an ongoing current infection. Five to 9 weeks after the infection started, a peripheral blood sample would show a high number of eosinophils. Children with iron deficiency anemia would have low blood levels of both iron and ferritin.

The goals are to treat ongoing infection and restore iron levels if deficient. There are medications that may be used to treat hookworm infection. These medications are effective only for the adult stage and not the different larval stages. Children two years of age and older may be treated with Albendazole, a 400 mg single dose given orally with a 33 to 100% cure rate. Alternatively, they may be treated with Mebendazole 100 mg oral chewable tablet given once or may be dosed twice a day for three days. This produces a 13 to 91% cure rate. Pyrantel pamoate may be used but has a lower rate of cure and higher risk of persistent infections.

Success rates are predicated on these medications only being effective in treating adult worms in the gastrointestinal tract. Larvae that have not developed into adults are not affected. Timing wise the larvae may develop into adults after treatment has been administered. This accounts for the variability in treatment success. Due to exposure, reinfections are common. Giving multiple doses may prove more effective in catching the time migrating larvae have developed into adults especially when incorporated into deworming programs. Rescreen feces four weeks after treatment has been completed to determine if there has been continued infection or if reinfection has occurred.

Children with iron deficiency anemia would be given iron supplementation 3–6 mg/kg/day divided into three equal doses for at least one month. It should not be given at the same time as multivitamins or calcium. An upset stomach may occur from the iron but may be minimized by giving Hershey kisses at the same time. The iron and ferritin (iron stored in the bone marrow) should be checked in 4 to 6 weeks. If levels are still low, continue iron supplementation.

There is an effective veterinarian dog vaccine for hookworm. Vaccination trials are underway for developing an effective human vaccination. To be effective, this vaccination would target both the adult stage and larval stages of hookworm. Current prevention measures include education about how hookworms are acquired, footwear to protect the feet, improved sanitation, better hygiene and safe water.

Hydatid Disease

Echinococcosis. Cystic Echinococcosis:
Echinococcus granulosus. Echinococcus multilocularis

Echinococcosis Hydatid disease, Cystic echinococcosis is caused by the dog and fox tapeworm *Echinococcus*. It causes slow growth of a hydatid metacestode cyst in intermediate mammalian hosts including humans. It may occur anywhere in the world but is more likely to occur in Asia, South America, North and East Africa, Southwest Europe, Canada, the United States, New Zealand and Australia. It is endemic in Uruguay, Chile, Southern Brazil, Peru, Argentina, the Mediterranean region, Central Asia, Northeast Africa and Western China.

In the United States it is found in Alaska, Arizona, California, New Mexico and Utah. As many as 5 to 10% of all people in Peru, Argentina, East Africa and China are infected with *Echinococcus*. There are two primary types of *Echinococcus, Echinococcus granulosus* and *Echinococcus multilocularis*. As many as 88% of all human cases worldwide are specifically due to *Echinococcus granulosus*. Risks factors are travel or living in areas where it occurs and exposure to dogs and livestock in these areas.

Echinococcosis is more likely to occur in rural communities where livestock are raised and graze in pasture areas. Sheep are at risk especially if they have close contact with guarding or herding dogs. *Echinococcus granulosus* infects over 1 million people. For its lifecycle it needs both an intermediate and a definitive host. The intermediate hosts are herbivores, grazing animals like buffalo, camels, sheep, goats, pigs, cattle and horses. They acquire the eggs of *Echinococcus* through grazing and pigs by eating infected feces. The intermediate hosts are required for some stages of parasite development. The definitive host, the one in which adult worms develop and produce eggs are carnivores, dogs and foxes as well as wolves that feed on the grazing animals or dogs that are fed the viscera of home butchered infected pigs, goats, sheep or cattle.

Echinococcosis may additionally be transmitted by flies, beetles and other insects. They transmit the parasite by feeding on or touching infested feces then touching food or water that is consumed by other mammals. Domesticated dogs and cats may become infected if they eat infected rodents. Eggs may be passed in dog feces and found on dog hair, paws and muzzles. Children and adults may acquire eggs by playing with these dogs. Infection may also occur from ingestion of salads, vegetables and uncooked fruits that are contaminated with *Echinococcus* eggs. It may also be acquired by handling contaminated soil or plants then direct transmission from the hands into the mouth. Trappers, hunters and anyone working with fox fur are exposed to *Echinococcus multilocularis* and at risk for alveolar hydatid disease. All mammals may serve as an intermediate host if they ingest *Echinococcus* eggs. Severe and fatal disease only occurs with infection in the intermediate not the definitive host.

The adult egg producing stage is found in the small intestines of carnivores. The carnivore is the definitive host and may be infected by hundreds of adult worms. Each worm may produce thousands of eggs every day. The eggs are in the last segments of the worm's body, the gravid proglottids which disintegrate and release eggs into the feces. These eggs are infective when passed in the feces and may remain infective for months up to years depending upon favorable environmental conditions. The eggs are in the soil and grass. When they are ingested by grazing animals, the intermediate host, eggs in the intestinal tract will hatch into an oncosphere. The oncosphere will penetrate the lining of the intestines, passing into the blood vessels and migrate to different internal organs. In the different organs, the oncosphere will develop into a fluid filled sac, the metacestode larval stage and is called the "hydatid cyst". Inside the hydatid cyst small vesicles called brood capsules bud from its internal lining producing the protoscoleces. New daughter cysts may also develop.

It may take up to 10 months after infection has started for the first protoscolece to develop. When this infected intermediate host is devoured by a carnivore, the protoscoeice is released and attaches to the intestinal lining. In 4 to 7 weeks, they will develop into mature adult worms. The adult worms are small ranging from 1 up to 7 mm in length. A single hydatid cyst may be several liters in volume and have thousands of protoscoleces. In the carnivore intestine each protoscolece may develop into an adult worm.

The *Echinococcus* cystic lesions may occur anywhere in the body of the intermediate host. Symptoms are the result of the location, size and degree of development and its effects on adjacent organs and structures. More than 90% will occur in either or both lungs producing alveolar echinococcosis and liver causing cystic echinococcosis. There are nine different subtypes of *Echinococcus granulosus* and *Echinococcus multilocularis*. Cystic echinococcus is caused by *Echinococcus granulosus* and alveolar echinococcosis is caused by *Echinococcus multilocularis*. It is the metacestode larval stage of each species that shows organ specificity. *Echinococcus multilocularis* metacestode will infect the liver then by tumor like growth extend or metastasize to the lung and brain.

Global estimates are that there are 2 to 3 million cases of echinococcosis, and most cases are cystic. It is most often asymptomatic for children and discovered incidentally when a CT scan, ultrasound or x-ray is done for another reason. Even though infection may occur during childhood, because the cysts are slow growing, 1 to 5 cm (a little less than 1/2 inch to nearly 2 inches) per year, diagnosis made from the development of symptoms may not occur until adulthood. Only 10 to 20% of hydatid cyst disease is diagnosed during childhood.

Before diagnosis, a cyst may spontaneously rupture, collapse or disappear. Only 10 to 20% of infections are diagnosed in those less than 16 years of age and those are more likely to involve the brain. Even a small cyst in the brain may cause significant symptoms. Liver cysts grow more slowly than alveolar cysts accounting for their delayed onset of symptoms and diagnosis at an older age. 40 to 80% of those with hydatid disease will have a single cyst in a single organ and 20 to 40% will have multiple cysts or multiple organ involvement.

It is estimated that there are around 18,000 new cases of alveolar echinococcosis each year. There is a high mortality rate for alveolar echinococcosis. If it is untreated or receives limited treatment the mortality may be as high as 90% 10 to 15 years after the initial diagnosis. By comparison the mortality rate for cystic echinococcosis is 2 to 4%. The lung is the most commonly involved organ for children. For adults, 70% of cases involve the liver, 20% the lungs and less frequently the heart, bone, spleen, kidneys and brain. Symptoms of lung involvement would be fever, shortness of breath, chest pain, chronic coughing and coughing up blood which occurs because of a cyst eroding into the lung tissue. It may perforate into the space between the lung and the chest wall, causing buildup of fluid in this space, a pleural effusion. This could cause the lung to collapse producing a pneumothorax.

Cystic echinococcus is usually asymptomatic unless rupture causes anaphylaxis (shock) or a cyst becomes infected, the cyst develops a connection to adjacent organs (fistula) or creates a mass compression effect on the organ or adjacent vital structures like nerves and blood vessels. If liver damage occurs there will be elevated liver enzymes from inflammation and elevated bilirubin. Bilirubin is a marker of impaired liver metabolism and jaundice. Recurrent cystic echinococcosis may occur after surgery due to rupture or leakage of cystic fluid releasing larvae which will grow into more cysts.

Early treatment for a cyst in any location may prevent cyst rupture. Cysts, even those that are contained will still cause chronic inflammation. They secrete immunosuppressive and other toxic products that may contribute to the development of malignant tumors and host damage. Liver damage and cyst rupture are the main causes of death. When cysts rupture, the release of toxic products into the bloodstream that affect blood vessels will lead to anaphylactic shock.

Rupture is most likely spontaneous but could occur as result of surgery or blunt trauma to the cyst area. Signs and symptoms of a cyst in the liver are liver enlargement, nausea, vomiting and upper abdominal pain. Cysts in the liver may cause liver damage, scarring and fibrosis. They may erode into surrounding channels and blood vessels or produce compression of the bile ducts that empty liver contents into the intestine. A cyst in the liver could rupture into the liver, gallbladder and biliary ducts. This would produce fever, jaundice, abdominal pain and vomiting. Liver cysts in time lead to liver failure and death. Rupture of heart cysts could cause embolism and clots that pass to the brain causing a stroke or lungs causing pulmonary embolism. Alternatively, cysts may become infected producing abrupt fever, abdominal pain and a high white blood cell count.

The presence of a cyst like mass and dog exposure in areas endemic for echinococcosis would support the diagnosis of cystic echinococcosis. A complete blood count (CBC) may have fewer than 25% eosinophils, a marker for allergies or parasitic infestation. Increased numbers of eosinophils may occur after rupture or leakage of a cyst. The gold standard and initial step for diagnosing a hydatid *Echinococcus* cyst is an ultrasound. However, a cyst may look like a malignant or benign tumor or other mass. It may be impossible to determine with certainty until other testing is completed. Small cysts and those in the lung and brain may not be detected by ultrasound. Other diagnostic radiology tests would be a CT or MRI scan. They are more accurate and sensitive. They would not only show the presence but also determine the state or condition of a cyst. Bone cysts may cause extensive bone erosion seen on these scans. Scans would show tumor like masses with characteristics of a central cavity. Similarly in the lungs, alveolar echinococcosis would produce the typical observed changes.

Serology blood testing may show antibodies to the *Echinococcus* parasite. Specific anti-echinococcosis antibody levels occur in the bloodstream 4 to 8 weeks after infection started. Early and inactive cysts may not trigger a significant immune response to produce a positive serology test. Similarly, a single cyst may not cause measurable antibody levels and a positive serological test. Cysts in the eye, bone, brain and those calcified stimulate no or low antibody production. If antibody levels are measurable, positive IgM titers are consistent with a current or recent infection and IgG titers mark an infection sometime in the past.

Liver cysts are more likely to produce an immune response and measurable antibody production than alveolar cysts. However as many as 10 to 20% of liver cysts and 40% of pulmonary cysts do not produce detectable antibody levels. PCR on biopsy or aspirated material from a cyst is more sensitive and may provide the definitive diagnosis.

A cyst may be "staged" based on features shown by ultrasound. Depending on the stage of the cyst, treatment may be through surgery, percutaneous aspiration, medications or by observation and watchful waiting. Cysts may calcify over time and become inactive. Surgery is the choice for large, infected cysts, cysts that are in certain organ locations or have a chance of rupture. Overall surgery is the treatment of choice if the entire cyst can be removed without spilling its contents because it results in a complete cure.

Surgery is also the preferred treatment for cysts in the brain, liver or lung, those secondarily infected or liver cysts larger than 10 cm. For alveolar cyst, usually the entire infected lung lobe is removed. Early diagnosis results in fewer unresectable lesions and radical surgery for alveolar echinococcosis. However, surgery may activate inactive cysts. Surgery for a liver cyst may result in removal of a lobe of lung or segment of the liver depending on the extent of the disease. Surgery is generally not an option for multiple cysts. Unfortunately, recurrent or continued disease is possible if other cysts were not detected and removed, or the cyst was only partially removed or leaked. It is recommended to continue a Benzimidazole for up to two years after surgery for both alveolar and cystic disease.

Cysts may have a needle inserted into them through the skin, percutaneous. The contents would be suctioned out and agents directly injected into the cysts to kill the parasite. A 95% ethanol or 20% hypertonic sodium chloride solution would be injected followed by aspiration in 15 to 20 minutes. These are toxic and kill protoscoleces in the cyst. Additionally specific medicines, Benzimidazoles may be injected at the same time and continued for up to 1 month.

If there are multiple compartments in the cyst which is possible, each one needs to be individually treated. This may be done to supplement or in some cases replace surgery but may allow leakage of cyst contents. This method has a lower rate of complications and disease recurrence with a shorter hospital stay compared to surgery. Leakage of cyst contents during or after the procedure may cause anaphylaxis or spread of the disease and development of additional cysts. It is not recommended for alveolar cysts.

Benzimidazoles, Albendazole and Mebendazole are the most effective drugs for treating echinococcosis cysts. They may be given before and after aspiration or surgery for cystic disease. They are indicated where surgery or aspiration is not possible for inoperable cysts or those with multiple cysts. Cysts in bones respond less to medicine compared to those in other sites.

Reports are that 10 to 30% of all those treated with Benzimidazoles are cured with complete, permanent disappearance of the cyst. 30 to 70% will have a reduction in cyst size and cyst related symptoms. Unfortunately, 20 to 40% do not respond favorably. However, these results may be a generous overestimation of the actual effect of Benzimidazoles. Relapses have occurred in 14 to 25% of those treated but usually respond well to retreatment.

Benzimidazoles are more effective for smaller cysts and may have limited benefit for those greater than 10 cm in size. They are given with fat rich meals. Albendazole has the best intestinal absorption and penetration into cysts. It produces the best results and is now the medicine of choice. It is the most commonly used medication even in children less than six years of age for alveolar echinococcosis. It may be given 10 to 15 mg/kg/day divided into two equal doses or 400 mg twice a day with meals. It must be given for a minimum of at least three and up to six months. Overall, it is well tolerated but may have a toxic effect on the liver and bone marrow. These are reversible effects when the medication is discontinued. It is recommended to have screening laboratory studies including a complete blood cell count and liver enzymes checked every two weeks for the first three months then monthly as long as therapy is continued.

Alternatively, Mebendazole may be used when Albendazole is not available. It may be given 40 to 50 mg/kg/day in three equally divided doses for

3 to 6 months. Benzimidazoles may be needed long-term for an inoperable cyst. Praziquantel and Nitazoxanide are ineffective for alveolar echinococcosis. Combining Albendazole with Praziquantel has been shown to be more effective than single drug therapy for treating hydatid disease.

The individual should be monitored carefully with an ultrasound and blood work for at least three years after completion of treatment. Long-term treatment with Albendazole is critical for those with active inoperable lesions or after surgery for *Echinococcus multilocularis*. It should be given for a minimum of two years for alveolar echinococcosis. Monitor these patients for at least 10 years for recurrence. For cystic echinococcosis it may be given at the treatment dose or up to 20 mg/kg/da divided into two doses for 4 to 5 years up to 20 years.

Liver transplantation has been done for those with end-stage disease. The diseased liver segment is removed, and the disease-free lateral areas are used for auto transplantation. However immunosuppressant treatment that follows transplantation may stimulate cysts in the liver or brain to grow.

There is a vaccination for cystic *Echinococcus* in sheep, the EG 95 vaccination. It produces effective protection after 2 doses. It may be used to protect other livestock from *Echinococcus*. There is no *Echinococcus* vaccination for people but human clinical trials of the EG 95 vaccination seems reasonable and warranted.

Liver Fluke

Fasciola
Fascioliasis
Fasciola buski
Fasciola hepatica (Sheep Liver Fluke)

Fascioliasis is a food borne illness of animals feeding on *Fasciola* contaminated vegetables. Infection preferentially occurs in cattle, sheep, goats, people, dogs, pigs, and rabbits. Fascioliasis has a worldwide distribution because of the geographical distribution of its snail host. It is estimated that worldwide 17 million people are infected with *Fasciola*. It has been reported in 81 countries including China, Taiwan, Indonesia, India, Nepal, Pakistan, Bangladesh, Thailand, Vietnam, Malaysia, Lao People's Democratic Republic, Bolivia, Brazil, Peru, Chile, Mexico, the Caribbean, the Netherlands, Portugal, Turkey, Iran and Egypt.

Fasciolia buski is found only in Asia and Africa. *Fasciola hepatica* has a nearly worldwide distribution because it adapts to changing environmental conditions and develops new hosts. The occurrence of infection in people in Mexico is reported to be between 2.9 and 13.3% and 0.6 to 1.75% in Pakistan. In parts of Bolivia the infection rate is 70%.

Fasciolia is trematode (fluke) acquired by ingestion of contaminated raw or undercooked vegetables grown in soil and also freshwater. Sources that lead to infection are contaminated plants including wild and cultivated freshwater plants, wild and cultivated plants grown in soil, foods and soups made from contaminated water, drinking beverages made from contaminated plants, drinking contaminated water and washing utensils and objects with contaminated water. Commonly ingested contaminated foods include watercress, water chestnut, water bamboo, water caltrop, radish, spinach, lettuce, salad vegetables and corncob. It may be transmitted in freshly prepared alfalfa and other vegetable juices. Vegetables grown on land may be contaminated when washed with contaminated water

Adult *Fasciola buski* worms are found in the duodenum and jejunum of the intestinal tract. They produce and release immature eggs in the stool. These eggs will mature and embryonate in water in 3 to 7 weeks. The miracidia hatch out of mature eggs and infect snails. In 4 to 6 weeks the miracidia will develop into cercariae in the snail. Cercariae are free swimming and will attach and form a cyst on the surface of aquatic plants forming the metacercaria stage. Animals and people become infected when they ingest a plant having the encysted metacercaria stage. In the gastrointestinal tract *Fasciola buski* metacercaria are digested out and over three months will develop into an adult fluke in the small intestines.

During their development over a 2-to-4-month period before juvenile *Fasciola hepatica* worms become adults they will pass through the intestinal wall into the abdominal cavity. From there they migrate to the liver. They burrow into the liver forming channels or tracks feeding on liver cells until in about 6 months after infection started, they reach the bile ducts. There they become mature egg producing adults. Adults may shed eggs from the liver and bile ducts for more than 10 years. Infection at other sites would be rare but possible. These other sites would include the pancreas, brain, eye, lung, skin and throat.

Estimates are that only 15% of all those with *Fasciola* infection are symptomatic. Symptoms depend upon the amount of parasites and damage caused by the parasite's toxic products produced and released by the worms. Symptoms may be identified as acute if lasting less than four months and chronic if persisting longer than four months. The adults in the intestines will also disrupt the production of intestinal enzymes and cause excessive mucus to be produced. Those with few parasites may have no symptoms. Alternatively, children may develop abdominal pain, bloating, poor appetite, vomiting, diarrhea and anemia. These symptoms are more likely with *Fasciola buski* which stays within the intestinal tract. Heavy infections with a high number of adult worms may result in malnutrition, significant inflammation of the intestines with ulcers, bleeding, abscess and scar tissue formation and perforation of the intestines or bile ducts.

Adults may migrate to the lower right abdomen and produce appendicitis type pain. The heaviest infections may additionally produce swelling of the abdomen, ascites, edema with swelling of the face and low-grade fever.

Adult worms range between 20 and 40 mm in size. From their size and numbers, they may produce obstruction and mechanical blockage of the gastrointestinal tract and bile ducts. This would prevent passage of contents within the intestines and trapping or sludging of bile in the gall bladder and bile ducts. For *Fasciola hepatica*, this may lead to jaundice, gallstones, cholangitis and scarring of the gallbladder. Other symptoms may develop depending upon the specific organs infected. With liver involvement, examination would show an enlarged tender liver located in the right upper abdomen area and a yellowish color to the skin and eyes, jaundice.

Definitive diagnosis is through visualizing eggs or adult worms microscopically in stool. Serology testing may be performed measuring IgG and IgM antibodies. Peripheral blood sample would show an elevated number of eosinophils. PCR analysis of stool would show *Fasciola* DNA. Endoscopic examination would show *Fasciola buski* adults in the intestines. With *Fasciola hepatica* infection, a CT or MRI scan would show cysts like clusters in tracts in the liver.

Treatment shortens the length of the symptoms and reduces the occurrence of complications. For children, the drug of choice for treatment of *Fasciola* is Triclabendazole. It is dosed on a single day 7.5 mg/kg twice a day after meals. It treats both adult, juvenile worms and their eggs. It produces a 100% cure rate. An alternative medication would be Praziquantel 25 mg/kg three times a day for one, two or three consecutive days. It produces a 100% cure rate. Measures of a complete cure and recovery would be that symptoms are completely resolved, no eggs are found in the stool, serology titers are decreasing, no eosinophils are seen in the peripheral blood smear and for *Fasciola hepatica*, an ultrasound or CT scan shows improvement with changes in the liver and bile ducts indicating healing.

There is no effective vaccination for the prevention of *Fasciola*. Key measures for prevention would include education about not ingesting raw or undercooked vegetables. Also, the availability of clean drinking water that may be used in food preparation and washing all utensils and surfaces is critical as well as proper sanitation measures.

Lung Fluke

Paragonimus
Paragonimus kellotti
Paragonimus westermani

Lung fluke is a pararsitic infection caused by the trematode *Paragonimus*. Infection begins with ingestion of raw, pickled or undercooked infected freshwater crab and crayfish. It will infect all mammals and has been recovered from people, mink, muskrat, opossum, coyotes, cats, dogs, lions, mongooses, wolves, leopards, boars, civets, raccoons, red foxes, gray foxes and bobcats. Different species of *Paragonimus* may infect different wild and domestic animals in different geographical areas.

In Asia the predominant species is *Paragonimus westermani* and in the Americas it is *Paragonimus kellotti*. It has a wide distribution and is found in China, South Korea, Philippines, Taiwan, Japan, Thailand, Vietnam, Laos, India, New Guinea, Cameroon, North and South America from Peru to Southern Canada, Venezuela, parts of Ecuador, Midwestern and Southern American states in the Mississippi River basin, Africa, Liberia and Nigeria. The only areas of the world that it has not been reported are Europe, Australia and Antarctica. Travelers, refugees and immigrants from endemic areas as well as imported contaminated food results in worldwide cases.

Estimates are that anywhere between several million up to 21 million people worldwide may be infected with lung fluke. The environment they live that supports the presence of freshwater crabs and crayfish, putting nearly 300 million people at risk for infection from *Paragonimus*. In certain parts of China, 10 to 28% of people have *Paragonimus* infection. The prevalence for children in India is nearly 52%.

Paragonimus has a complex lifecycle. Animals will ingest freshwater (ponds, streams, rivers) crabs or crayfish infected with the metacercaria encysted in their muscles, gills, legs and liver. Likewise, people may ingest raw, undercooked or pickled infected crabs or crayfish. During digestion in the intestinal tract the metacercaria excyst and are released. They pass through the wall of the intestines, usually the duodenum and travel to the abdominal cavity, brain, heart and lining of the chest wall. In 6 to 10 weeks, they mature into adult worms. The time from beginning of infection until eggs are produced is 60 to 90 days. In the lungs they release unfertilized eggs into the bronchioles, small airway channels of the lungs. These eggs are then coughed up in sputum and are either spit out into the environment or swallowed into the stomach and eventually pass in the feces. Only those adults in the lungs will pass eggs back into the environment. Adults at other body sites have no exit for their eggs.

In the environment the eggs require 2 weeks to develop and hatch the miracidia. Miracidia are motile and penetrate the snail body. In the snail the miracidia will undergo several developmental maturations forming the cercariae. The cercariae will be released into freshwater, seek out and penetrate the crab or crayfish. In the crab or crayfish, they will develop into the metacercaria and encyst in the gills, liver or muscle. When the crab or crayfish is ingested by a mammal, the metacercaria are digested out in the intestines and penetrate the abdominal wall. They migrate to different areas and mature into adults. Eggs produced in the lungs will pass back into the environment, completing the lifecycle.

Early and mild infections with few worms are usually asymptomatic. As worms mature and produce eggs, those in the lungs may cause coughing, initially dry then become wet. Chest pain, difficulty breathing and in time coughing up blood occur and mimicking tuberculosis. Lung symptoms may start 6 months after the onset of infection. A secondary pneumonia may develop. 10 to 20% develop fever. Metacercaria in the abdomen may cause abdominal pain, fever and diarrhea. Those that migrate to the brain will cause headaches, weakness, visual changes with possible blindness and seizures.

For the diagnosis, the clinician must have a high index of suspicion from the child eating raw, undercooked or pickled infected crabs or crayfish. The diagnosis is made by finding eggs in the sputum or feces. Bronchial washings of the lungs may provide a sample for microscopic examination for eggs. A complete blood count would have a high number of eosinophils. A chest x-ray may show signs consistent with pneumonia and cysts in the lungs. Serological tests would show IgG antibodies which would indicate infection but may not specify ongoing or acute infection at that time. Positive IgM antibody would indicate a current, ongoing or recent infection. Specific molecular tests, the PCR test and monoclonal antibodies are more specific for *Paragonimus* and would indicate ongoing infection. In certain select situations surgical removal of adult worms may be necessary for both improvement of symptoms and providing diagnostic material.

Paragonimus infection may be effectively treated with a three-day course of Praziquantel. It is dosed 75 mg/kg/day and divided into three equal doses. The cure rate after a three-day course of Praziquantel is 100%.

There is no effective vaccination for *Paragonimus*. Controlling *Paragonimus* in its different stages in animals, snails, crabs, crayfish and mammalian host is unrealistic. The key is education for people about proper cooking and not ingesting raw, pickled or undercooked crabs or crayfish. It is also important to thoroughly cook any animal that may have ingested infected raw freshwater crabs or crayfish.

Malaria

Plasmodium
Plasmodium falciparum
Plasmodium vivax
Plasmodium malariae
Plasmodium ovale
Plasmodium knowlesi

Over 150 *Plasmodium* species have been identified infecting mammals, birds and reptiles. There are five species that cause malaria in people, *Plasmodium falciparum*, *Plasmodium vivax*, *Plasmodium malariae*, *Plasmodium ovale* and *Plasmodium knowlesi*. Even today malaria is a critical health issue in different areas of the world. It is present in all hemispheres but more likely to occur in the Tropics and Subtropics, Sub-Saharan Africa, Latin America, Oceania and Asia. *Plasmodium falciparum* and *Plasmodium malariae* have a worldwide distribution. *Plasmodium ovale* occurs in Africa, Asia and Oceana. *Plasmodium vivax* is less likely to occur in Sub-Saharan Africa but is common throughout other areas of the world. It is the most common cause of malaria in Asia and the Americas. *Plasmodium knowlesi* occurs in clusters in Thailand, Singapore, Philippines, the Malaysian peninsula, Borneo and Myanmar.

Around 40% of the world's population lives in areas where there is active malaria. Estimates in 2017 were there were 219 million cases of malaria with 435,000 deaths. As many as 80% of all malaria cases and 90% of malaria deaths occur in Africa predominantly in children younger than 5 years of age. Compared to adults, children show malaria symptoms earlier and are more likely to have severe malaria disease. In 2020, it was estimated there were 241 million cases of malaria with 627,000 deaths in 85 different endemic countries with 95% of cases in Africa. Today there are as many as

2 million deaths primarily occurring in children in Sub-Saharan Africa due to *Plasmodium falciparum*. Overall *Plasmodium falciparum* causes the most severe cases and greatest number of deaths. Both worldwide travel and commerce have increased the exposure to malaria and along with immigration have resulted in it now occurring in new areas or areas where it had been successfully controlled.

Cumulative data shows there are approximately 1500 cases of malaria in the United States each year with these coming from travelers and immigrants from areas where malaria is active. As recent as the 1930s, malaria was a significant health problem in 13 Southeastern American states. In 2023, cases of *Plasmodium vivax* malaria were reported in the United States in Florida, Texas and Maryland in people who had not traveled outside the country. Mosquito traps in Florida recovered 1000 anopheles mosquitoes, transmitters of malaria, with three having malaria DNA in their gut from feeding on people with malaria.

Malaria is spread by the bite of infected female anopheles mosquitos that feeds from dusk to dawn. When a malaria infected mosquito feeds it transfers the sporozoite stage to humans. Over several hours the sporozoite spreads through the skin layers into the bloodstream. From there in 1 to 2 hours they may pass into the liver and multiply within the liver cells developing into the merozoite stage. Each liver cell may have 10,000 up to 30,000 merozoites. For *Plasmodium falciparum* and *Plasmodium malariae*, the liver stage may last 2 weeks. For *Plasmodium vivax* and *Plasmodium ovale*, the liver stage may occur quickly or remain latent in the hypnozoite stage for months to years before producing illness. Once produced, the merozoites are released into the bloodstream and enter into red blood cells. Inside the red blood cell, a wall is formed around the merozoite creating a vacuole.

The red blood cell merozoites develop into trophozoites then finally into schizonts over 24 hours for *Plasmodium knowlesi*, 48 hours for *Plasmodium falciparum*, *Plasmodium ovale* and *Plasmodium vivax*, and 72 hours for *Plasmodium malariae*. This correlates with the specific pattern for reoccurring fever seen with each species of malaria with recurring fever every two days with *Plasmodium falciparum*, *Plasmodium vivax* and *Plasmodium ovale*, recurring fever every 3 days for *Plasmodium malariae* and nocturnal fever occurring every day with *Plasmodium knowlesi*.

Feeding mosquitoes will ingest the infected red blood cells. In their midgut the parasite is released and forms gametes that fuse to make a zygote. These develop into ookinetes that burrow into the mosquito midgut wall.

These ookinetes develop into oocytes. The sporozoites are released from oocytes and over 1 to 2 weeks will migrate to the mosquito's salivary gland. Feeding of the female mosquito transfers sporozoites to the next host. Alternatively, malaria may be spread by needles shared by drug abusers, contaminated blood transfusions and infected organ transplants. A recommendation is to have a 1-to 3-month delay before travelers or immigrants from endemic areas are permitted to donate blood. This may still be inadequate because immigrants and travelers may harbor malaria for months to years before showing symptoms.

Malaria symptoms will follow with some variation depending upon which type of malaria is causing infection and the age and health of the infected person. There may be a delay of 12 up to 35 days or longer for symptoms to develop after an infected mosquito bite. Most malaria cases are due to *Plasmodium falciparum* which is estimated to cause 193.5 million cases each year and *Plasmodium vivax* reported each year to cause 14.3 million cases of malaria. *Plasmodium knowlesi*, *Plasmodium ovale* and *Plasmodium malariae* account for less than 5% of all malaria cases. The incubation period for *Plasmodium vivax* and *Plasmodium ovale* is 2 weeks. These forms may have relapses occur 2 to 3 years after an infection as a result of activation of residual latent, resting hypnozoites in the liver. *Plasmodium malariae* has an average incubation of 18 days. It will produce a low-grade symptomatic infection that may last for years.

Plasmodium falciparum and *Plasmodium malariae* have no dormant hypnozoite stage in the liver and therefore will not have relapses. It is the infected red blood cell stage that is responsible for the clinical symptoms of malaria. The general malaria symptoms are fever, chills, influenza-like symptoms with muscle aches and headache. The urine may have a dark, Coca-Cola color due to the presence of hemoglobin from the breakdown of red blood cells and is called "Blackwater fever". As a result of having multiple or ongoing infections with malaria, individuals will develop partial immunity and have a lowered risk of severe disease. Children, pregnant women and travelers to endemic areas or those who moved out of endemic areas and have no additional malaria infections may have low or no immunity. They would with reinfection be at risk for severe disease.

Plasmodium falciparum is the most severe form of malaria. It causes the most serious malaria symptoms and should be treated as a medical emergency. It may initially produce only mild symptoms but may rapidly progress and within 2 to 3 days of infection starting cause multisystem organ failure.

In addition to the general malaria symptoms. it may produce low blood count (anemia), low platelet count (thrombocytopenia), easy bleeding, liver inflammation with jaundice and kidney damage progressing to kidney failure.

Lung complications, "Malaria lung" will occur with severe *Plasmodium falciparum* infection causing fluid to fill the lung air exchange spaces, alveoli, leading to pneumonia and breathing failure. As the alveoli become filled with fluid, progressive breathing difficulties and breathing failure follow. Early signs of malaria lung may be blueness around the lips that spreads across the face and extremities and a dry cough that progresses to coughing up blood. Death may occur within 24 hours due to pulmonary failure.

Cases of severe malaria caused by *Plasmodium falciparum*, may develop brain damage, "Cerebral Malaria" producing a change in the level of consciousness and coma. They may have a stiff neck. The individual may develop seizures. For cerebral malaria the fatality rate may be around 18% due to brain swelling, cerebral edema, and blockage of the brain blood vessels impairing blood flow and oxygen delivery. In children who survive cerebral malaria, it will cause neurocognitive impairment with poor long-term reading skills. The fatality rate for uncomplicated *Plasmodium falciparum* malaria is 0.4%. For those with severe malaria the fatality rate is 15 to 30% with death occurring as soon as 3 to 8 days after the onset of infection. 80% of all malaria deaths occur in children younger than 5 years of age.

Plasmodium knowlesi has a high fatality rate in certain areas of the world and in severe cases may cause anemia, impaired, compromised kidney function and breathing difficulties. *Plasmodium vivax* is more indolent but twice as likely over time to prove fatal when compared to other types of malaria. Severe complications from malaria are the result of the infected red blood cells adhering to the lining of small blood vessels producing blockage. This will interfere with blood flow to the organs producing symptoms of oxygen and blood starvation. Stroke-like symptoms may occur with brain involvement.

The body in response to infection produces different inflammatory mediators called proinflammatory cytokines which also contribute to blood vessel damage. Malaria complications are more likely to occur in non-immune individuals who are susceptible to malaria or have lowered immune system activity. This would include children especially if less than 5 years of age, travelers to endemic areas who have not had malaria and pregnant women whose immune system function is already reduced.

Prompt identification, diagnosis and treatment especially for *Plasmodium falciparum* are critical for the outcome of malaria infections. Any traveler who has fever and is returning from an endemic area should be tested for malaria. The gold standard for diagnosis has been identifying infected red blood cells in a Giemsa-stained thick blood smear. This may initially be negative because infected red blood cells adhere to the lining of blood vessels and not be free-floating in the blood. Recommendations are to repeat a blood smear every 8 to 12 hours until the diagnosis is determined.

If there is not a heavy load or low amount of malaria parasites in the infection, there may be too few infected red blood cells to be seen in a blood smear. If the diagnosis is still uncertain, it may be worthwhile to run a PCR on the blood sample looking for malaria DNA. Additionally, *Plasmodium vivax* will only infect the red blood cell precursor call the reticulocyte, not the mature red blood cells cycling in the bloodstream.

Blood tests measuring IgG and IgM antibodies may be positive or negative depending upon the timing of collection. IgG antibody would signify a past malaria infection. A positive IgM antibody without a positive IgG antibody would be consistent with a current ongoing infection. If both IgG and IgM antibodies are positive, this may indicate a recent infection. Other more definitive tests on blood samples include a nucleic acid amplification test, NAAT and as already mentioned a PCR test.

There are a number of different antimalarial medicines that may be used. These include Chloroquine, Amodiaquine, Piperaquine, Sulfadoxine-Pyrimethamine, Malarone, Doxycycline, Mefloquine and Artemisinin derivatives. Selection depends on the specific type or species of malaria and the geographic area where malaria was contracted. It is best to check with the World Health Organization or the Centers for Disease Control about changing recommendations for treatment and patterns of antimalarial resistance.

Plasmodium falciparum is resistant to Chloroquine. Other types of malaria, *Plasmodium vivax*, *Plasmodium ovale*, *Plasmodium malariae* and *Plasmodium knowlesi* overall are Chloroquine sensitive with a few isolated pockets of resistance noted. Chloroquine is the first medication of choice to treat these infections. Severe malaria may require intravenous Artesunate as well as an oral medication. If secondary bacterial pneumonia or sepsis occur, an appropriate antibiotic is needed. For *Plasmodium vivax* and *Plasmodium ovale*, oral Primaquine is given to eliminate the hypnozoite liver stage that produces recurrence or relapses of malaria. There is a new drug Krintafel given as a single 300 mg dose in combination with Chloroquine to prevent relapses from *Plasmodium vivax*. It is approved for those 16 years of age and older.

Blood exchange transfusions have been part of the treatment for severe Malaria but are no longer recommended.

A critical step in prevention is considering factors that increase or promote malaria illness. Malaria is more likely to occur during the rainy, wet seasons. Man made environmental changes need to be carefully considered due to their positive and negative impact on the health and well-being of people. Damming of rivers and other water projects, changes in agricultural methods and deforestation may create new habitats for mosquitoes.

Reducing breeding areas for mosquitoes is a key first step in prevention. Mosquitoes will travel only short distances resulting in malaria outbreaks occurring around airports. Through the movement of travelers and immigrants, malaria may be imported from endemic to malaria free areas. Those infected may have and harbor malaria for months to years before becoming symptomatic.

Alternatively military personnel, forest and agricultural workers and hunters with no immunity moving into malaria endemic areas will increase the malaria susceptible population. Travelers to malaria endemic areas should take prophylactic malaria medication, use topical insecticides, stay in quarters that are air-conditioned or if not possible have screens in windows and use bed netting treated with an insecticide. Optimally apply a sunscreen agent to the skin before applying the DEET insect repellent product. Clothes to be worn during the trip may be prewashed with a permethrin detergent. This would serve as an additional deterrent for insects. When possible, avoid outdoor exposure during peak feeding time for malaria mosquitoes which lasts from dusk to dawn.

Malarone, Chloroquine, Mefloquine and Doxycycline have been used for prophylaxis for travelers to endemic areas. Malarone eradicates the liver stage of *Plasmodium falciparum* but not for *Plasmodium vivax*. When used, Malarone should be taken the same time each day during every travel day plus each day for seven days after returning from the trip. The other medications used for prophylaxis should be taken for four weeks after leaving the malaria endemic area to eliminate the merozoite stage as it passes into the bloodstream. These agents have no effect on the liver stage of malaria. Prophylactic antimalarial medicine may not be 100% effective, usually the result of not taking the medication correctly.

Certain ethnic populations in geographic areas have undergone genetic mutations making them more resistant to malaria infection. There may be mutations in hemoglobin producing modified hemoglobin S, C, E, or thalassemia. Changes may occur in red blood cell membrane shape or function, hereditary spherocytosis and xerocytosis or metabolic changes like the glucose 6 phosphate dehydrogenase deficiency protect against malaria infection. Certain ethnic groups, 2/3 of the black population, have a red blood cell type with no Duffy receptor on their surface. *Plasmodium vivax* uses this receptor for attaching to and initiating infection in red blood cells. This modification has made them resistant to *Plasmodium vivax* infection. *Plasmodium vivax* mutations have occurred allowing infection to occur in Duffy negative red blood cells.

A malaria vaccination has been developed. Mosquirix (RTS,S) has been developed from a sporozoite protein and produces short-term protection against this stage of malaria infection. It is a 3 dose shot series completed by 2 years of age. A fourth dose may be given which extends the protection by another 1 to 2 years. It is recommended for children living in malaria endemic areas. The initial protection is 74%. One year post vaccination the protection rate is 28% and drops to 9% five years after the vaccination was given. The vaccination is less effective in very young children. It will reduce the severity of symptoms but is not totally protective.

A second malaria vaccination has been developed, the R21 vaccination directed against a sporozoite protein. It is given as a shot with 3 doses, each dose given every 4 weeks followed by a fourth shot given 12 months after the third dose. It is cheaper and more available than the Mosquirix vaccination. With this vaccination children are more likely to have a febrile seizure. After the fourth dose it produces 75% protection over the next 12-month period.

There is a special monoclonal antibody designated C1543LS that protects against malaria infection. It is given intravenously and may be used for short-term passive protection. A second newer monoclonal antibody L9LS is in clinical trials. It may be given intravenous or subcutaneous, but higher dose intravenous is more effective. These have a high malaria antibody titer and are not a vaccination. They may have a time limited benefit being effective over six months. They work by coating sporozoites with an antibody which triggers an immune system response. The immune system will recognize and destroy these coated sporozoites. The use of a monoclonal antibody product may be an alternative for prophylaxis for travelers to endemic areas.

Additional vaccinations and approaches are needed that target different points of malaria transmission and stages of its development.

Pinworms

Enterobius
Enterobius vermicularis

Pinworms are common and endemic in Western countries including the United States. The last estimates were that there were 40 million infections in the United States in the 1980s. As many as 30% of the entire worldwide population has pinworms. It may affect all groups especially families and those living in close quarters. It is very common in young children, particularly those in kindergarten or living in institutions. They may produce few or no symptoms for most infected adults and children. There is an overrated hysterical concern by parents over their children being infested. First of all pinworms are specific for people and not spread by contact with pets or animals unless eggs are on their fur.

Secondly, we are all infested with pinworms but maintain a balance (commensal) in our system. If we develop an imbalance, there are more pinworms in our system than our system can handle, then symptoms may occur. The female pinworm is about 1 cm in length, a little less than 1/2 of an inch. Pinworms have a lifespan of about three months with only one month as an adult. The adults live in our large intestine mainly the cecum and the appendix. The males may live for about seven weeks and die after mating with the females. The females in turn die after they migrate down to the anus at night where they lay as many as 10,000 eggs. The eggs become infectious in about six hours. They will survive for about two weeks outside the human body. The eggs are ingested into our body through our mouth then hatch into larvae in the small intestines. They mature over the next month. The adults will repeat this cycle producing new eggs.

The peak occurrence for pinworm infestation is in children between five and 10 years of age. The predominant symptoms are in the evening. As we physically slow down, the worms become more active and move around causing evening stomachache. The females will crawl out the anus and lay their eggs. They may crawl and deposit their eggs in the vaginal area and on the scrotum. The protein slime layer they leave behind and their eggs may both create local irritation and contact dermatitis. This may lead to severe scratching and a secondary bacterial skin infection. Scratching may result in pinworm eggs under the fingernails and then putting hands into the mouth could lead to (auto) self-infection. As a result of the itching, infested children may have difficulty resting comfortably and have loss of sleep along with nighttime urinary accidents. Severe infestations are rarely seen in developed countries but may produce loss of appetite, weight loss and emotional irritability. Pinworm infections may also be associated with appendicitis.

Pinworm infestation is not from poor hygiene. Overcrowding may be the single most important factor in promoting its spread. The worms may be acquired by ingesting their eggs from salads, fruits and vegetables that have not been properly washed. Their eggs may be spread by children putting their hands, toys or environmental objects contaminated with eggs into their mouth. Contaminated fingernails from scratching their anus may serve as a source as well and perpetuate an infestation. If the eggs hatch on the anus, the larvae may enter the intestinal tract through the anus. Additionally, without hand washing with soap and water, hands may be contaminated after defecation even with using toilet paper. Pinworm eggs are ubiquitous and may be air-born and dust-borne, easily spread by air currents. This has been demonstrated by finding pinworm eggs over door thresholds and around windows in orphanages that have been closed for years.

It has been recommended for diagnosis of pinworm infestation to do the scotch tape test. The sticky side of scotch tape would be applied to the anal area when the child first arises in the morning. Then the tape should be folded over and taken to your physician for examination under a microscope looking for eggs. Unfortunately, most physicians' offices no longer have a microscope to do a visual inspection. Infected stool does not have eggs and there currently is no PCR or serology test to diagnose pinworms. Alternatively, you may see the adult worms around the anal area several hours after a child has fallen asleep. If a scotch tape test cannot be done or does not show eggs or pinworms are not seen around the anal area, a presumptive diagnosis may still be made by a child having redness around the anus, anal itching, disrupted sleep and abdominal discomfort early in the evening.

Measures to prevent pinworm infestation would be good handwashing and washing kitchen utensils frequently. Keep children's fingernails cut short to minimize scratching and transmission of eggs under the fingernails. Those with symptomatic pinworm infestation could sleep wearing tight fitting underwear, then change and launder the underwear first thing in the morning. This would minimize egg spread. Also, they could be bathed in the morning for cleansing any contaminated areas of their body. It is recommended that all household contacts and care givers, whether symptomatic or not receive treatment to minimize spread within a household. It has however been found that even after effective treatment reinfestation is common. It is usually only a matter of time before reinfestation occurs with most remaining asymptomatic.

There is an important distinction between reinfestation and symptomatic infestation. This speaks to the fact that we routinely take in pinworm eggs through our daily diet and activities. When treatment is needed, there are several different medications used for symptomatic pinworm infestations in children. Albendazole, 400 mg may be given as a single dose, but a second dose may be required. Mebendazole is recommended as a single 100 mg dose. Alternatively, Piperazine phosphate (4 grams) or pyrantel pamoate (11 mg/kg) may be given as a single dose. Piperazine works by paralyzing the worms so they may be passed in stool. Albendazole, Mebendazole and Pyrantel kill the adults but not eggs. A repeat dose of these medications may be given 2 to 3 weeks later to kill or eliminate adults hatched from eggs after the first dose was given.

It is recommended that all household and close contacts be treated. Since pinworms are more of a nuisance and create little health issue, it is most likely overkill and unnecessary to treat asymptomatic individuals in contact with a symptomatic child. Since there is a high likelihood that those treated will become re-infected, it would seem wiser to only treat symptomatic individuals. Additionally repeated doses of medicine may promote resistance and reduce or eliminate their effectiveness. These medicines may also cause toxic adverse side effects. Mebendazole may produce abdominal pain, diarrhea, hives, liver inflammation and low white blood cell count. Pyrantel may produce nausea, diarrhea, vomiting, headache, abdominal cramping pain, insomnia, loss of appetite, liver inflammation and skin rashes. Piperazine may produce blurred vision, nausea, vomiting, diarrhea, dizziness, drowsiness, headache, muscle weakness and tremors. These medications also vary for their availability and expense. For example, one dose of Mebendazole may cost $400.

River Blindness

Onchocerciasis
Onchocerca volvulus

Onchocerca is a filarial nematode spread by the bite of an infected Blackfly. Global estimates is there are around 37 million people infected with *Onchocerca* across 31 different countries. Onchocerciasis occurs in Cameroon, South Sudan, the Central African Republic, the Democratic Republic of the Congo, Yemen and the Amazon border region between Venezuela and Brazil. The Blackfly prefers to live and breed around fast flowing rivers and streams. Transmission of the disease by Blackflies is very inefficient and estimates are travelers need to be exposed repetitively over 12 months to become infected.

It is best known for producing the eye disease, "River Blindness" but may produce severe developmental disabilities and cognitive impairment in children. Children with *Onchocerca* infection may have brain inflammation resulting in epilepsy. This is more likely to occur in children between three and 18 years of age.

Children and adults will become infected through the bite of an infected Blackfly. The L3 larvae is introduced into the skin during the infected fly taking a blood meal. These L3 larvae mature into adults over the next 6 to12 month period. Females live in subcutaneous tissues or deeper muscles in a surrounding protective wall that forms a nodule. The male may travel between different nodules to fertilize the females. The nodules will contain both adult males and females. 10 to 15 months after infection begins, females will start to produce and release microfilariae. The microfilariae will migrate through the subcutaneous tissues. The microfilariae will live in the upper dermis of the skin, nodules and in the eye.

Those located in the skin will be taken in by the Blackfly during blood feeding. Within the first one to two weeks in the blackfly, the first stage L1 larvae migrate from the Blackfly midgut to the thoracic muscles. There it will go through 2 additional stages of development (molts) forming the infective L3 larvae. Infective L3 larvae will then migrate to the head and feeding apparatus (proboscis) of the Blackfly. From there it will be transmitted through additional Blackfly feeding. The microfilariae may be passed from an infected mother to their fetus through the umbilical cord connective tissue. Children may become infected early in life through biting of infected Blackflies.

The female worms may live between 9 and 14 years and have 9 to 11 reproductive years releasing 1000 to 3000 microfilariae each day. The microfilariae may themselves live around two years in the upper dermis of the skin, nodules and in the eye. When they die, they trigger a immune system response which may be severe in the eye and lead to blindness, "River Blindness". Disease of the eye and skin appears tp be a result of the host immune system activation and response to dead and dying microfilariae. Ocular damage would involve the retina, optic nerve and cornea. When alive, microfilariae are not very irritating to the body's immune system.

There seems to be an epidemiologic/geographic difference with eye infections and blindness occurring more likely in West African savanna areas and skin disease more likely in African forest areas. There may also be loss of skin pigmentation producing a pattern of "leopard skin". There may be intense itching and thickening of the skin. People living in endemic areas will have multiple adult worms, sometimes more than 60 and thousands of microfilariae in their skin.

Diagnosis may be accomplished through a PCR test on a nodule or upper dermis skin sample. It is possible to visualize microfilariae microscopically from a skin sample. Through a slit lamp examination of the eye, microfilariae may be directly visualized. Alternatively, a skin patch test with diethylcarbamazine in a lotion is applied to the skin. It kills microfilaria in the skin resulting in a rash developing in 24 hours indicating infection. An ultrasound may be done to visualize deeper seated nodules.

Onchocerca has bacteria, *Wolbachia*, that coexists in the worm. It produces specific factors and cofactors that are important for the adult worm survival and reproduction. Antibiotics that target *Wolbachia* will result in its death and subsequent sterility of the *Onchocerca* adult. Specifically, Doxycycline is given 100mg a day for 6 weeks. Ivermectin will kill the microfilariae in the skin and has a moderate effect on the adults. For those with a high microfilariae load, treatment and killing microfilariae will produce severe skin discomfort and itching. The general approach has been to give Ivermectin every three months. Ivermectin is dosed 150–200 µg/Kg orally for children weighing more than 15 kg. This oral dose may be repeated every 6 to 12 months. This dose will kill both adults and microfilaria in the skin.

The Blackfly is a daytime feeder. Take precautions to minimize biting during the daytime. Outdoors and if necessary, indoors wear long pants and long sleeves if there are no screens and only open-air living. Keep an effective repellent on exposed skin areas. Keep living quarters closed and use air-conditioning when possible. Clothes may be washed with a Permethrin product which maintains effective insect repellent affect for at least four additional clothes washings. There is no effective vaccination for *Onchocerca*.

Roundworms of Dogs and Cats

Toxocara
Toxocariasis
Toxocara canis **(Dog roundworm)**
Toxocara cati **(Cat roundworm)**

Toxocara has a worldwide distribution and infects millions of children and adolescents worldwide. It may be found anywhere dogs and cat pets coexist with people. It may be spread in the environment by stray dogs and cats. It is a roundworm of cats (*Toxacara cati*) and dogs (*Toxocara canis*). *Toxocara canis* may occur in dogs, foxes, coyotes, and wolves. It is estimated that globally there are 900 million domesticated dogs with 11.1% infected with *Toxocara*. Estimates are that 17.0% of all cats are infected with *Toxocara*. There is a higher rate of infection in puppies and kittens compared to older animals. Additionally, 19% of the world population, more than 1 billion and as many as 1.4 billion people are estimated to be infected with *Toxocara canis*.

Toxocara has been reported in more than 100 countries. In the United States it is estimated that there are 43 million dog owners owning a total of 63 million dogs. Children become infected through close contact with soil contaminated with infected dog and cat feces in playgrounds, public parks, beaches, sandboxes and poor hygiene. Analysis of city park soil samples shows that 17.4 up to 60.3% in Brazil, 14.4 up to 20.6% in the United States, 13.0 up to 87.1% in Europe, 30.3 up to 54.5% in Africa and 6.6 up to 14.3% in Asia are positive for *Toxocara* eggs.

Humans are accidentally infected through ingestion of *Toxocara* larvae infected raw or undercooked meat, beef, chicken, swine, lamb, rabbit, ostrich liver and ingestion of water contaminated with Toxocara eggs. The parasite cannot develop and complete its life cycle in these animals and humans. Most cases have been found to occur in France, Spain, Austria, Brazil, Argentina,

Korea, Japan, China, India, Tunisia, South Africa and the United States. The reported seropositive rate for children in certain areas of Nigeria is 80%, 37.7% in Africa, 34.1% in Southeast Asia, 24.7% in the Western Pacific, 10.5% in Europe, 8.2% in the Eastern Mediterranean, more than 20% in certain parts of Mexico and 22.8% in the Americas. The seropositive rate for children in the United States ranges between 5 and 15%. It is more likely to occur in areas that have a higher number of pet, stray and feral dogs and cats.

Dogs and cats become infected by eating meat of infected animals that do not complete the parasite life cycle or by ingesting soil contaminated with embryonated eggs. Ingested embryonated eggs or encysted larvae are taken into the gastrointestinal tract and hatch in the small intestines. In dogs and cats, the L3 larvae of *Toxocara canis* and *Toxocara cati* will invade the intestinal wall. They pass to the liver and then into the bronchial tubes and trachea. From there they are coughed up and swallowed through the esophagus back into the intestines. There they develop into adult worms that may only live for 4 to 6 months. They will produce noninfectious, non-embryonated eggs that are released with feces into the environment. Each female adult worm may produce and release 200,000 eggs daily. In the soil eggs will undergo maturation and become embryonated, forming infective eggs that may survive for months to years in a favorable warm and moist environment. Older animals may have the larvae encyst in their tissue during migration. Female dogs and cats when pregnant will have these larvae excyst, reactivate, cross the placenta and infect the developing puppies and kittens (transplacental infection).

The highest rate of infection with *Toxocara canis* is in puppies. They may become infected before birth with larvae passing transplacental. They may also become infected through taking their mother's milk. Estimates are that 50% of all puppies have acquired infection in utero, before they are born and have a positive test by two weeks of age. 70% of all puppies have positive test for *Toxocara canis* by 12 weeks of age. Compared to puppies, kittens are less likely to become infected with Toxocara cati. However, like puppies they may become infected before they are born as well as through feeding on their mother's milk.

For animals including people that are not the natural host for this parasite, *Toxocara* cannot complete its life cycle. For these animals the L3 larval form is released in the small intestines and penetrates the intestinal wall. It then migrates through the blood vessels to different organs throughout the body. *Toxocara* disease may be specified by its tissue migration pattern and preferred organ for infection. Larva in tissue cannot undergo any additional development. *Toxocara* produces different substances that reduce its triggering of the host's immune system. This helps it to evade attack by the host's immune system. However as noted, *Toxocara* larvae cannot complete their life cycle in people. Larva will become walled off in cysts. Cysts may survive for up to 7 years in people but eventually die in the infected tissue. This will trigger an immune system response. Damage results from the combined effects of mechanical damage produced by migrating larvae, inflammation from larval death and the immune system's response to that specific trigger. The immune system will form a protective wall or "granuloma" around the dying or dead larvae. The tissue damage that occurs is irreparable.

Types of *Toxocara* illness

Visceral Larva Migrans: *Toxocara* larvae migrate through tissues of the viscera, this includes solid and hollow organs in the abdomen. It may involve the heart, lung, kidney, muscles and liver. The liver is the most commonly infected organ for people. Symptoms of Visceral Larva Migrans are related to its migration through tissue and selected organs for infection. It may cause fever, nausea, vomiting, loss of appetite, wheezing, abdominal pain, enlarged tender liver, elevated eosinophil count and elevated liver enzymes. There may be a rash, itching, breathing problems, chronic cough, eczema, muscle aches, inflamed heart and blood vessels and swollen and sore subcutaneous fat. Involvement of the heart is rare but will lead to heart inflammation, heart weakening, heart failure and death. Visceral Larva Migrans is more likely to occur in children 2 to 7 years of age and is associated with heavy or repeated infections.

Ocular Larva Migrans: Occurs from larvae migrating into the back of the eyeball. Eye damage, retinal disease and blindness may result from the direct effect of the larvae on the eye and from the larvae dying from the host immune system response. There may initially develop blurry vision and light sensitivity. Specific eye damage will produce uveitis, retinitis, choroiditis, endophthalmitis and glaucoma. An abscess may develop in the eye. There is no increase in the white blood cell count or the number of eosinophils. Ocular Larva Migrans occurs in older children and adolescents.

Neurotoxocariasis: Symptoms are the result of migration to and persistence of larvae in the central nervous system. It may be caused by both *Toxocara canis* and *Toxocora cati*. There may be signs of brain inflammation with encephalitis, myelitis, meningoencephalitis, seizures and cerebral vasculitis.

These may prove to be fatal. Infected individuals may also have neuropsychiatric symptoms like anxiety, learning and memory impairment and signs of a neurodegenerative process.

Covert Toxocariasis: Is due to prolonged migration of larvae through the body which may last for years. Symptoms may be body aches especially the limbs, sleep problems, headache and loss of appetite. Other symptoms overlap with Visceral Larva Migrans, fever, abdominal pain, nausea and vomiting with swollen lymph nodes and an enlarged liver. It may produce an elevated eosinophil count due to prolonged tissue inflammation and trigger an immune system response with elevated markers of inflammation, the sedimentation rate and C reactive protein.

Toxoacara cati is more likely to cause more severe disease in people than *Toxocara canis*.

The gold standard for diagnosis of Toxocara would be identifying larvae microscopically in biopsied granulomas. A PCR test on a biopsied granuloma would show Toxocara DNA. A biopsy would be obtained only in the most severe cases. The next best option is serological testing looking for the presence of IgG and IgM antibodies against *Toxocara*. However, Neurotoxocariasis and Ocular Larva Migrans may have negative serology results. The presence of only IgG antibodies signifies that at some point in time infection did occur. It does not indicate an ongoing infection.

Adult *Toxocara* worms are not found in the human intestines. There would be no *Toxocara* eggs in stool for screening purposes. The best way to diagnose Ocular Larva Migrans is with an eye examination visualizing granuloma in the eye. Nonspecifically for other types of *Toxocara* disease a peripheral blood sample would show an elevated eosinophil count and markers of inflammation for specific infected organs (heart muscle, liver) may be elevated. An ultrasound, CT or MRI scan of the brain or liver would show granulomas.

Mild infection may require no treatment and be self-limited with recovery in up to 2 years. If treatment is needed, the preferred antihelminth agent is Albendazole given 10 mg/kg/day divided into two equal oral doses for five days. Ocular involvement is treated with Albendazole for 14 days. Neurotoxocariasis may be treated for 4 weeks with a recovery rate of 78.9 and 8 weeks of treatment with a recovery rate of 81.3%. A maximum dose is 400 mg twice a day. It is preferred because it has better tissue penetration compared to other anthelmintics. Other agents are not as effective or have more adverse side effects. Every case of Visceral Larva Migrans and Neurotoxocariasis is treated with Albendazole. Ocular, brain and heart involvement would also receive prednisone 0.5 to 1.0 mg/kg/day to reduce inflammation. To preserve vision, surgery, cryotherapy to remove a granuloma may be required for severe cases of Ocular Larva Migrans. If epilepsy occurs in those with Neurotoxocariasis, specific medicine for a seizure disorder is needed.

There is no effective vaccination for *Toxocara*. Direct contact with puppies or kittens is not a risk factor for acquiring *Toxocara* because the eggs they pass have not been in the soil to mature. These eggs are not embryonated and not infectious. However, at times pets may have embryonated eggs on their fur they have picked up from the soil. It is important to pick up and properly dispose of dog feces. Maintain good health of pets and have them dewormed per their veterinarian's direction.

Avoid common outdoor areas that are likely to be contaminated with dog and cat feces. General preventive measures are to not eat unwashed vegetables and fruits or raw or undercooked liver and meats. Thoroughly wash or cook all vegetables and fruits with clean water. Assure meats have been cooked at the appropriate temperature to destroy any *Toxocara* larvae. Thoroughly wash and disinfect all surfaces, cutting boards and utensils used to prepare meats. Good hygiene with effective handwashing helps to reduce acquiring *Toxocara*.

Schistosoma

Schistosomiasis
Schistosoma mansoni
Schistosoma haematobium
Schistosoma japonicum

Schistosomiasis is a widespread disease found in tropical and subtropical areas of the world. Depending on the area of the world, it is the second or third most common and important parasitic disease for children after malaria with its impact on public health and socioeconomic development. It is a waterborne parasitic disease caused by the *Schistosoma* blood flukes. Industrial development and dam construction creating man-made reservoirs and irrigation systems contribute to environmental changes promoting it's intermediate host snail population. Significant factors for people are inadequate sanitation and unsafe, not clean water. Population growth, global migration, holiday travel and adventure directed tourism have put unsuspecting travelers at risk for schistosomiasis and spread schistosomiasis to developed countries.

There are six different species of *Schistosoma* that may infect humans, but only three types are significant, *Schistosoma haematobium*, *Schistosoma japonicum* and *Schistosoma mansoni*. The World Health Organization estimates that it occurs in 79 different countries in Africa, Southeast Asia, the Middle East, South America and Caribbean with 229 million people worldwide infected with schistosomiasis. 91% of infected individuals reside in Africa. Countries of concern and interest are Kenya, Mali, Nigeria, Zimbabwe, Uganda and Cote d'Ivoire. Other areas and countries that have schistosomiasis are the Nile River valley in Egypt and Sudan, Iraq, Iran, Yemen, Saudi Arabia, Mallorca, Corsica, Suriname, Brazil, Venezuela, Southern China, Indonesia, the Philippines, Lao People's Democratic Republic, Cambodia, Dominican Republic, Martinque, Guadeloupe and Saint Lucia.

As many as 60% of all African children are infected with *Schistosoma*. Other estimates are that nearly 80% of children 4 months to six years of age who live in endemic areas have *Schistosoma* infection. Children may remain infected and untreated for several years. These infections may become chronic and have disease progression. If infections are long-term, the risk of bladder cancer, liver damage from hepatic periportal fibrosis (scarring) which may cause high blood pressure in the liver (portal hypertension), bleeding blood vessels in the esophagus and enlarged liver and spleen, infertility and susceptibility to HIV infection are all increased.

Health problems from schistosomiasis are more likely to occur in individuals living in endemic areas who have continued infection from repeated chronic exposure from using and bathing in contaminated water. Tourists and travelers with a more limited accidental contact with infection are at a lower risk of health problems. Their limited exposures may be from scuba diving, fishing, waterskiing, rafting, wading or swimming in contaminated fresh-water lakes, canals, springs, rivers and streams that are near tourist destinations. Unfortunately, there is no easy way to determine if the water is infected. The combination of so many infected people worldwide and favorable environments for the parasite to exist lead to it being a significant risk factor for both travelers to and individuals who live in these areas.

A favorable environment and presence of the appropriate snail hosts are all that are needed for water contamination and infection to occur. All ages will become infected ranging from babies as young as 4 months of age to all adults. In addition to people, *Schistosoma japonicum* may also infect dogs, cattle, water buffalo, pigs and rodents. These animals may contribute to expanding fresh-water contamination and *Schistosoma* transmission. Through their contamination of water, rodents are an important reservoir and significant source of infection for other animals and people.

Various programs have been underway to educate people in ways to minimize their risk of infection. These measures include mass drug administration to the entire populations in areas where there is a high occurrence of schistosomiasis and education as far as avoiding contaminated waters for bathing and recreation. However, this information is generally not shared and provided to tourists. Exposures of infants and babies may be indirect through these waters taken back into the home for bathing. The burden or number of worms in an infected individual is a direct result of the frequency of exposure to contaminated waters.

Certain specific species of snail are the intermediate host in contaminated waters. Infective cercariae emerged from infected snails. They are released into the water and with contact to exposed skin will penetrate the skin and initiate infection in people. A hives rash may develop within hours up to 1 to 12 weeks at the site of cercarial penetration of the skin. It itches and may be transient lasting for only several up tp 48 hours. Cercaria pass through the bloodstream to the lungs and finally reenter the bloodstream to pass to the bladder (*haematobium*) or liver (*mansoni, japonicum*). In the portal, liver veins (mansoni and japonicum) and bladder blood vessels (*haematobium*) the immature worms (Schistosomula) mature into the adult worms in 4 to 6 weeks. Next they migrate to their final destination. The adults are 7 to 20 millimeters (1/4 to 3/4 inch) long. They live on average 3 to 5 years but may live as long as 30 years.

Unlike other trematodes, Schistosomes have different sexes. The adult male and female worms of *Schistosoma haematobium* live in a peri vesical (bladder) blood vessels. The liver (portal) blood vessels and blood vessels in the intestinal lining of the large and small intestines (mesenteric) are the site for adult *Schistosoma japonicum* and *Schistosoma mansoni* flukes. They feed on the host's blood and regurgitate waste and debris back into their host's blood. The most severe lesions are found in the large intestines and rectum.

The adult flukes mate and deposit eggs in the capillaries of the infected organ. Eggs from the female *Schistosoma haematobium* pass into the bladder and are excreted in the urine. Eggs for *Schistosoma mansoni* and *japonicum* pass into the intestines and are excreted in the feces. An adult female may produce 300 to 500 eggs a day. Once the eggs pass into fresh water they hatch into the miracidium, the free living motile first stage larva.

The miracidium will infect specific fresh-water snails. After about 30 days in the snails the miracidium develops into the sporocyst which ultimately develops into cercaria. In the end, this process produces hundreds to thousands of cercaria which are released into the water. In 4 to 6 weeks after infection started, they begin leaving their snail host. They must contact a suitable host and penetrate the skin in 12 to 24 hours.

The rash history and timing of the fever may be important clues for travelers who have returned home. Other symptoms may occur anywhere from weeks, months or even up to years after a primary infection. They occur as result of the body's immune system response to *Schistosoma* eggs causing areas of inflammation, granulomas and scarring in the liver, intestines, bladder and lungs. The severity of symptoms is the combined result of the intensity of infection, number of worms, and the body's immune system response.

Typically, there is an abrupt, sudden onset of nonspecific symptoms, abdominal tenderness and pain, blood in the urine or stool, headache, cough, hives, shortness of breath, body ache, fatigue and diarrhea. Up to two thirds of those infected may develop night-time fever, "Katayama fever" 2 to 8 weeks after infection started. Cardiac symptoms include heart inflammation, pericarditis, myocarditis and heart rhythm abnormalities are unlikely but possible.

Nervous system, brain or spinal cord symptoms are more likely to occur from *Schistosoma mansoni* infection. Nervous system symptoms are the result of eggs and migrating worms in the brain and spinal cord. This may produce headache, blurred vision, weakness, numbness, dizziness, impaired or altered speech, seizures and unstable standing or walking. These may occur 3 weeks after other symptoms. Chronic symptoms are due to the immune system response to egg migration. There is granuloma formation and scarring. Those with chronic *Schistosoma japonicum* infection are more likely to have a tumor like expanding brain mass and seizures. The tumor is an expanding granuloma. Spinal cord Schistosomiasis is more likely with *Schistosoma mansoni* and causes lower back pain, pain in the lower legs and lower leg weakness or numbness. Paralysis may occur from eggs and granulomas at a certain level in the spinal cord.

Katayama syndrome may occur with the initial *Schistosoma* infection but is more likely to occur with chronic infection. It may occur 14 to 84 days after the first *Schistosoma* infection. Symptoms are cough, headache, nighttime fever, achiness, and abdominal tenderness. Similarly, Katayama fever usually occurs with the first infection but may occur in those chronically infected. It is an immune system mediated hypersensitivity reaction to immature migrating worms and highly immunogenic eggs. With the first-time infection, most individuals recover uneventfully in 2 to 10 weeks. However, some develop serious illness with weight loss, diarrhea, abdominal pain, shortness or difficulty breathing, and enlarged liver. It may also present as acute appendicitis with eggs producing obstruction of the appendix opening.

A complete blood cell count will show an increased number of eosinophils. An increase in this cell type is a nonspecific response seen with allergic reactions and parasitic infections. There may also be iron deficiency anemia. *Schistosoma haematobium* infection may produce blood in the urine. Depending on the species, diagnosis may be made by observing *Schistosoma* eggs in the stool or urine. Identifying the eggs in the urine or stool is still considered the "gold standard" for diagnosing Schistosomiasis. Alternatively, measuring antibodies made against the parasite may be through Hemagglutinin and ELISA serology blood tests. Results are more accurate when both types of serology tests are performed and done at a minimum of at least two months after the last exposure and opportunity for infection. Travelers are optimally screened 3 to 6 months after they return. Serology tests may remain positive after treatment. False negative results may occur due to a low burden of infection. Polymerase chain reaction tests (PCR) are more specific and selective and may detect small amounts of *Schistosoma* DNA or micro-RNA in urine, blood or stool. Rectal or bladder biopsy may show eggs in these tissues.

Imaging studies may be done to better assess the extent of *Schistosoma* disease. An ultrasound could evaluate liver, spleen and urogenital damage from infection. A chest radiograph could show lung involvement and bronchial and pulmonary lesions. CT and MRI scans of the brain and spinal cord would show lesions if present.

The medicine of choice to treat schistosomiasis is Praziquantel (PZQ). It is effective only against adult worms. It will paralyze and kill the adults but has no effect on the immature developing worms or eggs. It may be used to treat schistosomiasis in individuals as young as four years of age. There is no scientific information for its use in those one to four years of age but when used in this population it has been found to be safe with no adverse effects. It is available as a 600 mg tablet scored in 4 parts making it possible to individualize the dose and give 150 mg, 300 mg, 450 mg, or the entire tablet 600 mg. The tablet may be crushed making it easier for children of all ages.

For *Schistosoma japonicum* infections, Praziquantel is given 20 mg/kg per dose for a total of 3 doses. A dose is given every 4 to 6 hours. For neuroschistosomiasis, give Praziquantel for a total of six days. For the other Schistosomes, the total treatment is only two doses given in one day. Treatment is extended to three days for individuals having seizures secondary to brain granulomas. These cases need to be observed in the hospital during the treatment phase. For children with heart disease, they likewise should be monitored closely during administration of the medicine.

Corticosteroids may be added to the treatment when there is brain involvement (neuroschistosomiasis) or bronchial and pulmonary lesions to reduce the reaction to killed adult worms. Corticosteroids are given as a single dose of 1.5 to 2.0 mg/kg/day and should be used for 3 to 4 weeks then gradually tapered and weaned over another 3 to 4 weeks. Anticonvulsants may be needed to treat a seizure disorder from brain involvement. Neuroschistosomiasis if not aggressively and properly treated may be fatal. The goal is to treat neuroschistosomiasis early with Praziquantel and corticosteroids. Surgery may be considered to remove granulomas. For those with spinal cord lesions, estimates are that 65% recover fully or with minimal deficits. They recover more quickly when given steroid treatment. The optimal treatment combines both corticosteroids with Praziquantel. If untreated they are more likely to die from secondary infection. For travelers, treat with Praziquantel at least 6 to 8 weeks after their last potential infected fresh-water exposure.

Drug treatment with Praziquantel does not prevent reinfection. Praziquantel acts in concert with the host immune system. It may not kill all the worms with a single treatment. It has been observed that those with a heavy worm burden will have impaired brain function with lower cognitive test results and educational scores. To minimize brain damage from infection, medicine must be given early. It produces improvement for both verbal and speed of short-term memory. The *Schistosoma* cure rate with 1 treatment ranges between 63 to more than 90%. Retreatment may be required in 4 to 12 weeks and produces a cure rate of 95 to 100%. This helps to improve the overall health status. Treatment reduces damage produced from infection and reinfection and promotes improved immunity which may reduce both the occurrence and injury from reinfection.

It has been observed that children with schistosomiasis have a sub optimal response to vaccinations. This may be the result of the direct effect of the parasite and chronic infection interfering with the immune system activity or a result of the overall compromised, poor, weakened health status from infection. There are several *Schistosoma* vaccinations in development targeting the different species. A vaccination is considered effective if it reduces worm infection by 75%.

A question is whether vaccinations developed for schistosomiasis be given only to those who are not or have never been infected and what about those who are already infected? It is unknown if a vaccination would help to reduce complications from chronic infection, reduce the occurrence of reinfection and eliminate transmission by those already infected. It is speculated that the combination of an effective vaccination with continued treatment of entire populations with Praziquantel may be effective in eliminating it as a public health problem.

There is a concern that retreating entire populations with Praziquantel will contribute to the development of drug resistance. A single simultaneous administration of both vaccine and Praziquantel may reduce or eliminate the need for repeated treatment of entire populations or individuals. The hope would be that one cycle of this combination of an effective vaccination and Praziquantel would make it unnecessary for repeated drug administration and the potential for Praziquantel resistance.

Strongyloides

Strongyloides stercoralis

Strongyloides is a soil transmitted, skin penetrating nematode. It is more resistant and found throughout the world in temperate, tropical and sub-tropical areas including Southeast Asia, Cambodia, Thailand, Laos, Latin America, Spain, Sub-Saharan Africa, North America and parts of Europe. Strongyloidiasis is endemic in the Southeastern United States, the Appalachian region as far north as Kentucky with an estimated prevalence of 4% in Eastern Kentucky. Estimates are that worldwide 350 million people are infected with *Strongyloides*. Refugees, travelers and immigrants from endemic areas may import the disease. Dogs may also be infected with *Stronglyloides stercoralis* and a source of infective larvae in the soil.

Unlike other helminths, it is unique in that it has the ability to re-infect its human host, auto infection. Eggs may undergo maturation into infectious larvae during passage through the gastrointestinal tract and may then penetrate the large intestine wall or perianal skin. It may be passed from person to person by exposure to fresh infected human feces by those in close quarters or by skin contact with infected feces in the soil. It has been reported in children playing in infested outdoor areas with exposed skin, bare feet and hands and those attending day care. Because of the potential for self, auto infection, infection with *Strongyloides* could continue in the same person for decades.

Alternatively, eggs that pass into the soil will develop into filariform larvae. These larvae may be orally ingested and develop in the gastrointestinal tract. However most primary infections will occur from the filariform larvae in the soil penetrating exposed skin. They then pass through veins into the lungs. There they leave the blood vessels and enter the air exchange spaces (alveoli). The larvae are eventually coughed up and swallowed into the gastrointestinal tract where they might into adults. The females embed in the duodenum and jejunum of the small intestines and release eggs.

In the gastrointestinal tract these eggs will hatch and mature into their rhabditiform larvae in the soil mature into adults. Females are fertilized by males, eggs are then produced and released into the soil. The rhabditiform larvae hatch from the eggs. This stage then matures into the infective filariform larvae and waits for a host. Rhabditiform larvae remaining in the gastrointestinal tract mature into the filariform larva. The filariform larvae may penetrate the anal mucosa, reenter the circulation and restart the cycle.

Symptoms may be bloating and abdominal pain after eating as well as new onset heartburn and gastroesophageal reflux disease not caused by lying down. Irritable bowel symptoms may occur with alternating diarrhea and constipation. Nausea, vomiting, fever and anal itching may occur. The worms, due to their small size produce little lung inflammation and damage during that stage of migration. However, pneumonia could develop. Once the worms burrow into and pass through the skin they may leave a serpiginous (red) track that itch called larva currens. In chronic infections there may be hives or pimples on the abdomen or extremities showing an allergic sensitization to the parasite.

For those with a healthy, normal immune system, most infections including those chronic are asymptomatic and detected only after finding a high number of eosinophils in the blood. The lungs may become inflamed due to larval migration causing cough, shortness of breath and wheezing. If larvae penetrate the wall of the intestines, they may take bacteria along producing bacteremia, bacterial infection in the bloodstream and meningitis, infection into the brain. Septic shock and bleeding may develop with bruising around the belly button. If complications develop to this extent, there is a fatality rate of 35 up to 100%. These severe complications are more likely to occur if the person is immunosuppressed, receiving corticosteroids or elderly.

Microscopic examination of a thin blood smear would show an elevated number of eosinophils. It may take several weeks after infection has started to detect larvae in the stool. Egg excretion is intermittent and may pay multiple stool microscopic examinations to detect the parasite. Serologic testing may be more definitive using an enzyme linked immunosorbent assay (ELISA) but these early tests were not specific for *Strongyloides* and could detect other helminths. Newer ELISA tests are nearly 100% accurate for *Strongyloides* IgG antibody detection but only indicate infection at some point in time. A PCR test may be used to detect small amounts of *Strongyloides* specific DNA. Nucleic acid amplification tests (NAAT) have an increased sensitivity targeting specific DNA segments of *Strongyloides*.

Ivermectin is the drug of choice for *Strongyloides*. It targets both adults and larvae. A single dose of Ivermectin 200 ug/kg has been recommended to treat *Strongyloides*. A maximum dose of Ivermectin for children between 15 to 24 kg (33–55 pounds) would be 3 MG; those 25 to 35 kg (55–77 pounds) would have a maximum dose of 6 mg; those 36 to 50 kg (79–110 pounds) would receive a maximum dose of 9 mg; those 51 to 65 kg (112–143 pounds) would receive a maximum dose of 12 mg; those 66 kg or more (145 pounds) receive a maximum dose of 15 mg. Albendazole 400 mg orally twice a day for 3 to 7 days or Thiabendazole 25 mg/kg orally twice a day for 3 days has been used. Their comparative cure rates are for Ivermectin between 74 and 84%, Albendazole 48% and Thiabendazole 69%. The alternatives to Ivermectin are not as effective and produce more adverse side effects. A two-day course of Ivermectin 200ug (0.2 mg)/kg as a single dose each day may be more effective producing a 93% cure rate.

If *Strongyloides* has disseminated and spread outside the gastrointestinal tract then 14 or more days of Ivermectin is recommended. It has been given in the rectum or as an intramuscular shot in the leg or arm. For disseminated disease, Albendazole or Thiabendazole would be added to Ivermectin. Albendazole would be given 400 mg orally twice a day. Thiabendazole is dosed on two consecutive days with those weighing less than 13.6 kg (30 pounds) would receive 25 mg; those weighing 13.5 to 22 kg (30–48 pounds) would receive a maximum dose of 250 mg per dose; those weighing 23 to 34 kg (51 to75 pounds) would receive a maximum dose of 500 mg per dose; those weighing 35 to 45 kg (77–99 pounds) would receive a maximum dose of 750 mg per dose; those weighing 46 to 56 kg (101–123 pounds) would receive a maximum dose of 1000 mg; those weighing 57 to 67 kg (124–147 pounds) would receive 1250 mg as a maximum dose; those weighing more than 67 kg (147 pounds) would receive a maximum of 1500 mg. Medication will produce a cure but unfortunately due to environmental exposure *Strongyloides* reinfection is common. Vaccinations for *Strongyloides* are in the developmental phase. Today elimination of *Strongyloides* is through improved sanitation, proper disposal of human feces, clean drinking water and improved hygiene.

Toxoplasma

Toxoplasmosis
Toxoplasma gondii

Toxoplasma gondii is a ubiquitous protozoan parasite. It is one of the most common parasites that infect people. Estimates are that approximately 2 billion people up to 1/3 of the world population are infected with *Toxoplasma*. It naturally infects cats and other warm-blooded mammals, pigs, chickens, sheep, goats, lambs and people. Feral swine are an important source of *Toxoplasma gondii*. In the United States feral swine are found in at least 39 states with a population estimated to be around 5 million and growing every day. Testing shows that 17.7 up to 28.4% of all feral pigs in the United States are positive for *Toxoplasma gondii*. In the United States feral pigs are most likely found in the South and Midwest.

Worldwide estimates are that 17.6 up to 55% of all feral swine are infected with *Toxoplasma gondii*. They may acquire *Toxoplasma* through cannibalism of other infected animals alive or dead or through vegetation containing cysts. Comparative numbers show that 2.7% of confinement raised domestic pigs in the United States are infected with *Toxoplasma gondii* compared to 50 to 100% for pasture or free-range pigs.

Toxoplasmosis has been reported in France, Australia, Poland, Brazil, Guyana, Malaysia, French Guiana, Central America and the United States. It occurs more often in countries where raw meat is consumed. In certain areas of the world, 50 to 80% of people are infected with *Toxoplasma*. Estimates are up to 54% of those living in France, Latin America or Sub-Saharan Africa are positive for *Toxoplasma*. The *Toxoplasma* infection rate in Europe may be between 30 and 63%. In the United States, it is estimated that 8.3 up to 30% of the entire population is infected with *Toxoplasma* with the highest rate in the Northeast and lower rates in the South, Midwest and West. The incidence in the United States has been decreasing over the past several decades.

Indoor cats that do not hunt and are not fed raw meat but eat dry or canned processed cat food are unlikely to have *Toxoplasma gondii*. 62 to 80% of outdoor and feral cats are infected with *Toxoplasma*. Cats become infected by ingesting birds, rodents or other small mammals infected with *Toxoplasma* cysts (containing infectious bradyzoites) or anything contaminated with feces from infected cats. The eggs or cysts will undergo transformation and development growing into adult worms. Infected cats usually remain asymptomatic but in one to two weeks after infection started will excrete large amounts of noninfectious *Toxoplasma* oocytes (eggs) in their feces ranging from 100,000 up to 10 million each day. These oocytes develop 2 protective layers forming the oocyst which remains viable in the soil, sandbox, litter box or garbage for months to years. Oocysts are only shed by the definitive host cats in their feces. They are resistant to freezing for up to 18 months. It takes 1 to 5 days up to 2 weeks in the soil for cysts to develop infectious sporozoites.

When oocysts are ingested by the warm-blooded intermediate hosts, sporozoites are released from the cysts and penetrate the intestinal lining. There sporozoites develop into tachyzoites. Tachyzoites will migrate to different tissues and transform into the bradyzoite stage which surrounds itself with a protective wall, it "encysts" and is protected in the host tissue.

People may become infected with *Toxoplasma* by ingesting undercooked or raw meats infected with *Toxoplasma* cysts or by direct ingestion of food or water contaminated with oocytes or oocysts. In different parts of the world, 3 to 35% of pork, 7 to 60% of lamb and 0 to 9% of beef are infected with *Toxoplasma* gondii. Oocytes may be carried to food through flies or cockroaches. They may also be on the fur of dogs. Depending on the stage ingested, if the cysts are ingested from infected meat then bradyzoites are released from cysts in tissue or muscle. If cysts are taken in orally, sporozoites are released in the intestinal tract. Sporozoites will transform into tachyzoites and pass through the different developmental stages.

The tachyzoites multiply in the gastrointestinal tract then spread through the bloodstream throughout the body. The tachyzoites will grow and destroy surrounding tissue. The tachyzoites circulate for 3 to 10 days before transforming into bradyzoites which will form resistant cysts in tissues. Tachyzoites are killed by the body's immune system response. Cysts may form as early as seven days after infection started and remain for life in muscle or tissues of the infected animal or person.

Toxoplasma is rarely spread by blood transfusions or organ transplantation. Women infected with toxoplasmosis have a more difficult time conceiving and a higher rate of miscarriages. *Toxoplasma* may be spread from a pregnant woman to her developing baby, a condition called transplacental infection. Estimates are that in the United States 15% of all childbearing age women are positive for *Toxoplasma*. Comparatively in Canada estimates are 20 to 40% of all women of childbearing age have *Toxoplasma*.

Early in pregnancy there is a lower rate of actual transplacental transmission. There is some protective mechanism in place. The rate of transplacental transmission is estimated to be 10 to 17% in the first trimester, 22 to 40% in the second trimester and 65 to 68% in the third trimester. *Toxoplasma* infected women without treatment have a 20 to 50% rate of passing this infection to their fetus. In the United States estimates are that between 400 and 4000 children are born with congenital toxoplasmosis each year but the true occurrence is unknown because most babies are asymptomatic at birth.

The effects on the fetus are more devastating the earlier in pregnancy infection occurs. Transplacental infection in the first trimester may result in more severe disease and lead to fetal death. Second trimester infections may produce Sabin's tetrad of symptoms (hydrocephalus, brain calcifications, seizures and chorioretinitis) and third trimester infections are typically asymptomatic. These effects include a small baby with growth retardation, premature births or fetal loss, eye infection, chorioretinitis, brain lesions with cognitive and motor deficits causing intellectual disability, hearing loss and liver and lung inflammation. Neurologic and ocular disease are more severe in early transplacental infected babies. If undetected during pregnancy, 90% of *Toxoplasma* infected babies will have no symptoms at birth while others have signs of infection with a rash, a low platelet count and seizures.

Three different subtypes of *Toxoplasma* have been identified. They may vary in the severity of their symptoms. Most individuals infected with *Toxoplasma* remained asymptomatic. For the 10 to 20% who become symptomatic, they may have mononucleosis or influenza symptoms with a low-grade fever, swollen lymph nodes, chills, sweat, headache, muscle aches, sore throat, rash and malaise. Two percent may develop eye disease with chorioretinitis, loss of central vision or blindness due to autoimmune inflammation. Infection with certain subtypes of *Toxoplasma* in individuals with a genetic susceptibility may cause depression, suicidal thoughts and attempts or other mental illnesses.

The incubation period, delay between acquisition of infection and onset of symptoms may be 5 to 23 days. Symptoms and at times severe symptoms are more likely to occur in people who have an altered or impaired immune system and the *Toxoplasma* subtype producing infection. Severe symptoms would include heart damage, myocarditis, lung inflammation pneumonitis, brain inflammation, encephalitis and in the most extreme situations, death. Estimates are more than 90% of pregnant women who are acutely infected with *Toxoplasma gondii* show no signs or symptoms or if become ill with influenza-like symptoms but recover spontaneously.

Diagnosis of toxoplasmosis would be through measuring antibody levels. IgM antibodies are the first antibodies made and become measurable in 5 days to several weeks after infection started. A single positive IgM antibody may be a false positive test and needs to be tandem with a positive IgG as markers of ongoing *Toxoplasma* infection. Repeat the serology test in two weeks checking for a positive IgG antibody matched with a positive IgM titer. IgG antibody may first be detected in 1 to 2 weeks after infection started and peaks in 12 weeks to 6 months. Once present, IgG antibodies may persist for life. If on repeat testing the IgG antibody is still negative, the IgM test is most likely a false positive, the result of a cross-reaction with another trigger. A blood sample would have an increased number of lymphocytes with a cell type called atypical lymphocytes. Liver enzymes may be slightly elevated.

Microscopic examination of a fine needle aspirated cyst would show bradyzoites. Fine needle aspiration of an infected lymph node would show tachyzoites. A PCR test on the biopsy material would show *Toxoplasma* DNA. For those with eye involvement, an eye examination would show chorioretinitis. In the United States and Western Europe, 35% of all cases of chorioretinitis are due to *Toxoplasma*. Signs of chorioretinitis are blurred vision, light sensitivity. visual floaters, optic nerve damage and loss of central vision. On examination the liver and spleen would be enlarged and tender. A CT scan of the brain for a congenital/transplacental infection would show scattered calcifications.

Most individuals with toxoplasmosis require no treatment. If symptoms are severe or persistent, or there is evidence of damage to vital organs, treatment should be started to stop the damage. Treatment does not eradicate the cysts from the body but treats the tissue migratory phase. All infected fetuses and infected newborns should be treated even if they have no symptoms. They may at some time develop symptoms including early onset autism spectrum disorder while other deficits could be delayed until adolescence.

Infants should be treated for one year. They would receive Pyrimethamine 2 mg/kg/day (maximum 25 mg) orally divided into two equal doses for two days, then 1 mg/kg/day (maximum 25 mg) a day for two or six months, then decreased to 1 mg/kg/day (maximum 50 mg) on alternate days, Monday, Wednesday and Friday. It is also given concurrently with Sulfadiazine 50 mg/kg/day (maximum 4 grams) orally twice day with Leucovorin 5 to 10 mg orally on Monday, Wednesday and Friday. Pyrimethamine and Sulfadiazine work synergistically.

Spiramycin 1 gram taken orally every 8 hours may be given to pregnant women to minimize vertical spread to their fetus. It treats only the woman and does not cross the placenta. If she acquired *Toxoplasma* infection longer than 6 months before becoming pregnant, no treatment is recommended. If a fetus has a positive amniotic fluid PCR in the second or third trimester, treat the pregnant woman with Pyrimethamine and Sulfadiazine which would also treat the fetus. If the fetus becomes infected in the first trimester just give Sulfadiazine because Pyrimethamine will cause birth defects. Early treatment of a fetus with transplacental toxoplasmosis is effective in preventing organ damage and long-term complications. Alternative treatments for children and adolescents may include using Bactrim (Trimethoprim/Sulfamethoxazole) or Clindamycin.

There is no effective vaccination for *Toxoplasma*. Prenatal screening in areas of high *Toxoplasma* infection is critical. Keys for prevention are through education about risk factors and how the infection is acquired. Wear gloves when gardening or changing a cat litter box for cats that spend time out-doors or changing an uncovered sandbox. Avoid stray cats and stray kittens. Wash uncooked fruits and vegetables before eating and only drink safe water. Field dressing, butchering and handling raw meat of feral pigs and other game increases the risk of exposure for sport and game hunters. They should wear gloves. Be mindful that free range swine has an increased risk of being infected with *Toxoplasma gondii*. Do not taste meat before cooking. Diligent hygiene measures should be taken with proper cleaning with soap and water of cutting boards, utensils, knives and sink tops that may contact raw meat and vegetables.

Appropriate cooking of meats includes using a meat thermometer and heating the meat thoroughly to 152.6°F (67°C) for at least four minutes. More specific recommendations are for beef, lamb, veal and steaks to cook at least 145°F (63°C). Pork, ground meat and wild game are cooked at 160°F (71°C) and poultry at a minimum of 165°F (74°C) or preferably higher at 179.6°F (82°C). Use a food thermometer to ensure the proper cooking tem-perature has been reached. If meats are to be served rare, as a precaution the recommendation would be to freeze the meat at 10.4°F (–12°C) for several days before serving. Alternatively, another suggestion is cooling and freezing infected meat at 8.6°F (–13°C) for three weeks. Refrigeration and microwave cooking do not kill *Toxoplasma*. Other ways of preparing or preserving meats, curing, smoking and drying do not kill *Toxoplasma* cyst.

Trichinella

Trichinosis
Trichinella spiralis

Trichinella is a nematode roundworm acquired by ingestion of raw or under-cooked infected meat. It has a worldwide distribution and is found on all continents except Antarctica. It is estimated that 11 million people worldwide are infected with *Trichinella spiralis*. It usually occurs in small family sized outbreaks. As many as 30% of all people in certain parts of China are infected with *Trichinella*. The overall prevalence of infection is unknown. It has been reported in France, Italy, Poland, Romania, China, Thailand, Mexico, Argentina, Bolivia, Turkey, Vietnam, the United States, Japan, New Guinea, Thailand, Taiwan, Cambodia, Tanzania and Lebanon. In the United States it is reported in Kentucky, Iowa and the Southeastern states. There are nine different subtypes or species of *Trichinella* that may infect people with seven of them causing illness or disease.

In the United States, 30% of all human cases of *Trichinella* come from ingestion of infected, undercooked pigs and wild boar. Home raised and home slaughtered swine are a more common source than those commercially harvested. Home raised swine are more likely to be fed garbage or slaughtered animal parts, or those through free range ingesting Trichinella larvae. Wild pigs and game animals are a significant source especially for hunters that dress and eat their game. Other sources of *Trichinella* are deer, pigs, foxes, dogs, cougars, rodents, horses, bears, wild boar, moose and walrus. They become infected through carnivorous activity or ingesting larvae left on vegetation.

In the United States the feral swine population is estimated to be 5 million and growing rapidly. They have been found in at least 39 states and present a risk for both domestic and free-range pigs in unsecured areas. Feral and free-range domestic pigs will exhibit cannibalism and also eat carcasses left in the field from hunters. These are additional important sources for acquiring *Trichinella*. The significance of feral pigs as a source of *Trichinella* is supported by information that shows 3%, and in some areas as high as 5.1% of all feral swine in the United States, nearly 20% in Vietnam, 0.1% in Slovakia and 0.7% of pigs in Switzerland have *Trichinella* infection as demonstrated by positive antibody titers.

Infection begins with the ingestion of raw or undercooked meat or meat products that are infected with *Trichinella* larvae. The infected meat contains *Trichinella* larvae in protective cysts. In 2 to 7 days after exposure to stomach pepsin gastric acids, larvae are digested out of the cyst. Over 10 to 28 hours the larvae will undergo four transformations and mature into male and female adult worms that burrow into the intestinal wall. For up to five weeks, female worms produce and release larvae, then they die. The larvae penetrate the intestinal wall and pass through the bloodstream to heart, lung, brain, kidney and striated muscles (muscles that move like skeletal and heart muscle). The larvae will form a protective wall, encyst, in muscle cells. Some types of *Trichinella* do not form a protective wall.

In skeletal muscle cells, the larvae are provided nutrition that supports their growth and development. The larvae cause minimal damage to the muscle cels. Larvae with and without a protective cyst wall may remain viable for years before they calcify and die. When other organs are infected like the heart, brain, lungs, and kidneys, *Trichinella* larvae will produce cell inflammation, organ failure and death.

The severity of symptoms correlates with the number of ingested larvae. The adults in the intestines may initially cause abdominal pain, nausea, vomiting and watery diarrhea, the enteric or intestinal phase. The second wave of symptoms occurs 1 to 6 weeks after ingestion of infective larvae when they enter and pass-through different tissues. During the migratory phase there may be fever, weakness, swelling around the eyes and face, achiness, fatigue, hives and redness and hemorrhage in the whites of the eyes. The muscle may have tenderness, pain, swelling and weakness. These symptoms peak 2 to 4 weeks after infection started. Muscle pain is more likely to occur in the upper body, neck, shoulders and forearms versus calves in the lower extremities. There may be eye pain and difficulty with vision. Cough, shortness of breath and skin rashes with difficulty swallowing may occur. Symptoms may resolve around 10 days after they started.

Infection of the brain and nervous system, neurotrichinellosis, may cause headaches that are worsened by movement, body weakness, blindness, deafness, change in behavior and personality, seizures, unsteady walking and paralysis. Individuals with neurotrichinellosis survive but may have neurologic symptoms persist.

Liver inflammation may affect protein metabolism and liver function. Death overall is rare from trichinosis but may occur from an irregular heart rhythm occurring in the second week of the illness or weakening and failure of the inflamed and damaged heart muscle. Weakening of the breathing muscles with breathing failure or pneumonia, kidney inflammation and failure and brain infection, meningitis or encephalitis may all result in death.

Diagnoses would include evaluating a number of different parameters. A peripheral blood smear would show an increased and at times a massive number of eosinophils which peaks 3 to 4 weeks after infection started. The eosinophil count may reach 20 to 90%. Specific muscle enzymes, creatine phosphokinase and lactate dehydrogenase would be elevated. These are nonspecific changes, not unique for *Trichinella*. More specific testing would include measuring antibodies to *Trichinella*. These would become positive three weeks after ingestion of the contaminated meat and may remain positive for months. A confirmatory muscle biopsy could be performed on accessible cysts and be evaluated for its contents. A PCR test on biopsy material would show *Trichinella* DNA.

Mild infection with *Trichinella* does not require antiparasitic medications but is treated with pain and fever control measures. The optimal time for treatment is in the first several weeks after infection has started when only gastrointestinal symptoms are present. There is no effective treatment once muscle encystment has occurred. Mebendazole would be given 5 mg/kg orally twice a day for 5 to 6 days or 200–400 mg given orally three times a day for three days then 400–500 mg three times a day for 10 days. Mebendazole has been shown to be effective in eliminating adult worms from the intestinal tract. An alternative would be Albendazole, 400 mg orally twice a day for 8–14 days. It may be a better choice for treating pediatric patients. Prednisone 30–60 mg/day may be given for 10 to 15 days to reduce inflammation then taper over 2 to 3 weeks.

There is no effective vaccination for *Trichinella*. Effective prevention hinges around education that pigs are the most likely source of *Trichinella* infections. Backyard and free-range swine continue to be a source especially in developing countries. There may be a specific cultural approach for raising swine and consumption of raw or undercooked swine. It is important to keep livestock separated from wild or feral animals. Free range and feeding animals garbage or scraps of slaughtered animals should be discouraged.

Proper preparation of meat is key in preventing people from acquiring *Trichinella*. Meat should be cooked at a minimum temperature of 131°F (55°C) or higher until the pink fluid or flesh are not visible. The suggested parameters for cooking pork would be: 132°F (55.6°C) for 15 minutes; 136°F (57.8°C) for three minutes; 142°F (61.1°C) for one minute; 144°F (62.2°C) instantaneously. A cooking probe should be used and inserted into the meat to assure the proper temperature has been attained. Freezing is only effective for infected pork. Freezing is not effective for other *Trichinella* infected meats. Recommendations for freezing include 1°F (–15°C) for three or more weeks, 0°F (–17.8°C) for 106 hours or –5°F (–70.6°C) for 82 hours. Different recipes for curing meat will use salt, fermentation, different temperatures and drying times. These methods are not 100% effective in eliminating *Trichinella* larvae. The USDA has established standards for preparation and safety of potentially infected *Trichinella* meats.

Whipworm

Trichuris
Trichuris trichiura
Trichuris suis

Worldwide more than 430 million people are infected with whipworm. It is most common in areas of Asia, Africa and the Americas that are depressed or in poverty. School age and preschool age children are more likely to have and also have the heaviest burden, (numbers) of whipworm. The adult whipworm lives in the colon, preferably the cecum for one to two years. Males may be a little longer than females at 30 to 56 mm and females 30 to 50 mm, both between 1 to 2 inches. They will mate and the female produces and releases 3000 to 20,000 eggs into the feces each day. Eggs pass into the soil and for their continued development require specific environmental conditions, high humidity, warm temperatures and sandy soil. After 10 to 14 days and up to three weeks in soil with the right conditions, they mature and become infective. People become infected by ingesting contaminated foods that have been grown in egg infected, contaminated soil. In the stomach the L1 larvae hatch, pass into and penetrate the intestinal lining, molt and release an immature adult worm.

The immature adult worms pass into the cecum and large intestine (colon) where they develop into mature adults. The adults will embed into the wall of the colon. They insert their whip-like anterior end into the colon wall. They secrete enzymes and a protein which helps with their digestion. They may live one to three years in the host. It generally takes three months after ingestion for the worm to pass through the different stages reaching the mature adult stage and produce eggs. The eggs may be detected in the stool. Mild infection with *Trichuris* may produce mild or no symptoms but cause slowed, delayed growth.

High level of infection may cause colon inflammation, colitis involving the entire colon from the ileum to the rectum, from the first to the last part of the large intestines. *Trichuris* is a major cause of colitis and infection driven inflammatory bowel disease. There may be signs consistent with irritable bowel disease with chronic abdominal pain, diarrhea and bleeding. Large numbers of worms may cause dysentery like symptoms with mucus in the bowel movement and rectal bleeding. As result there may be significant weight loss, iron deficiency anemia, rectal prolapse and tenesmus. Chronic infection may cause severe malnutrition leading to delayed and impaired brain (cognitive) and body growth.

Intentional seeding the human intestines with *Trichuris suis* (pig whipworm) ova was considered as a potential treatment for irritable bowel syndrome. It would alter immune system activity and block the pathological immune system response that contributes to irritable bowel disease. Overall, to date, no benefit has been observed in those with ulcerative colitis or Crohn's disease after receiving *Trichuris suis* ova.

Diagnosis is by observation of characteristic eggs by microscopic examination of feces. A PCR test would show *Trichuris* DNA. A serology test would show a positive IgG with old or recurrent infection and IgM indicating an ongoing infection.

A single dose of oral Albendazole or Mebendazole produces a 25 and 33% cure rate respectively. Recommendations especially for heavy infections are to orally treat daily with Albendazole 400 mg for 3 to 7 days or Mebendazole 100 mg twice a day or 500 mg daily for 3 to 7 days. For prevention, use a combination of Albendazole and Oxantel pamoate. Alternative treatment may be through combining Albendazole with Ivermectin 200 µg/kg/day. This combination has been shown to have a better cure rate. In areas of high endemic disease, it may be beneficial for regular repeated mass drug administration, treating an entire population to reduce the prevalence and adverse effects from *Trichuris* infection. There is no vaccination for *Trichuris*.

www.ingramcontent.com/pod-product-compliance
Lightning Source LLC
Chambersburg PA
CBHW071716170526
45165CB00005B/2031